Annals of Gay Sexuality 2015

The Contemporary HIV Zeitgeist

www.annalsofgaysexuality.com

Smart and incendiary texts & images exploring current issues in gay men's sexuality.

Editors
Marcus Greatheart
Robert Birch

Art Direction
Pan

Contributors
Joshua Barton
Robert Birch
Pablo Cáceres
Wilson Copland
Wes Fanelli
Marcus Greatheart
Michael Horwitz
Francisco Ibáñez-Carrasco
Mischief
Pan
Grahame Perry
Lore Schmidts
Simon Sheppard
Michael V. Smith
Eric Sneathen
Navid Tabatabai
RM Vaughan

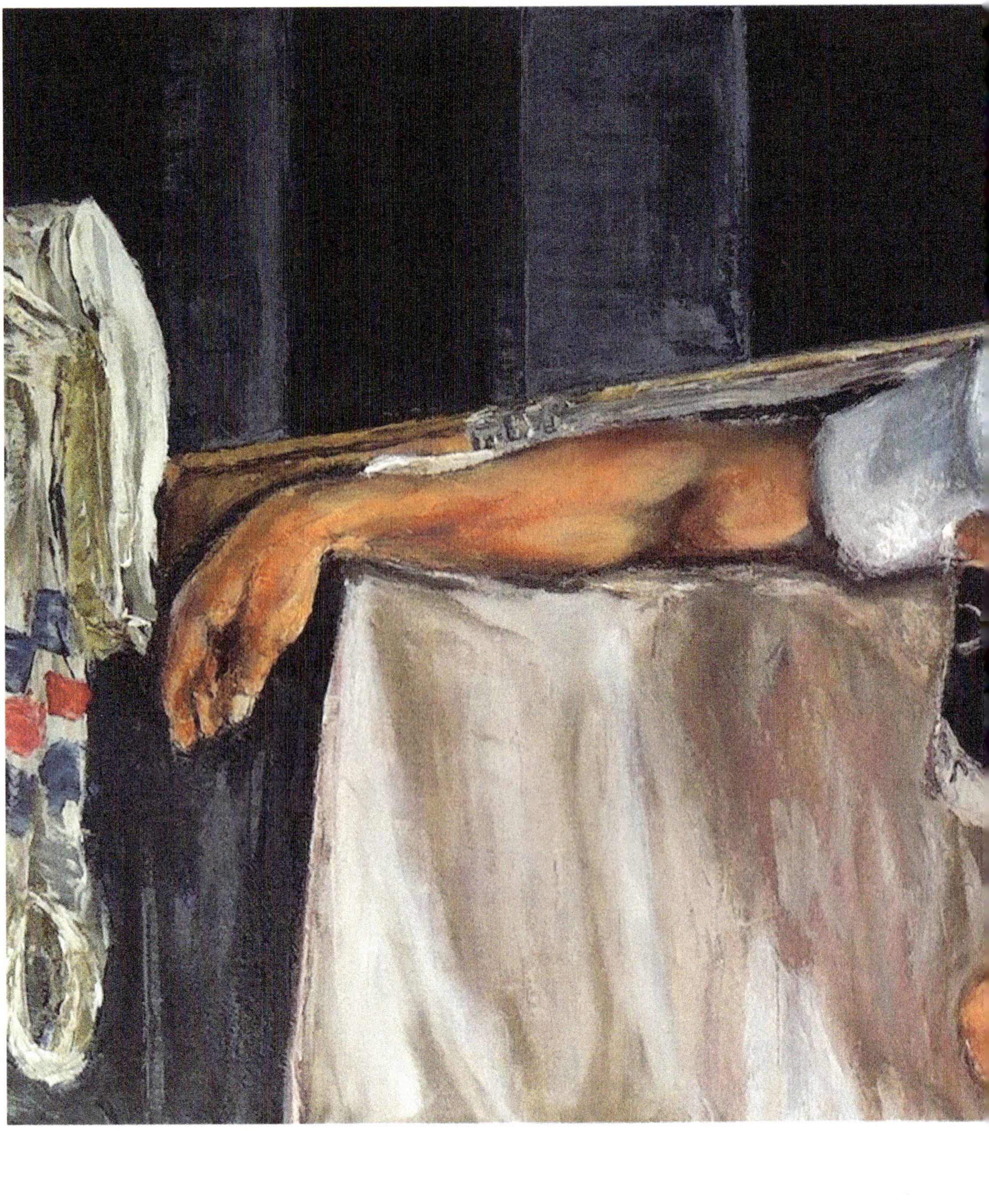

ABOVE:

Time Out | Lore Schmidts

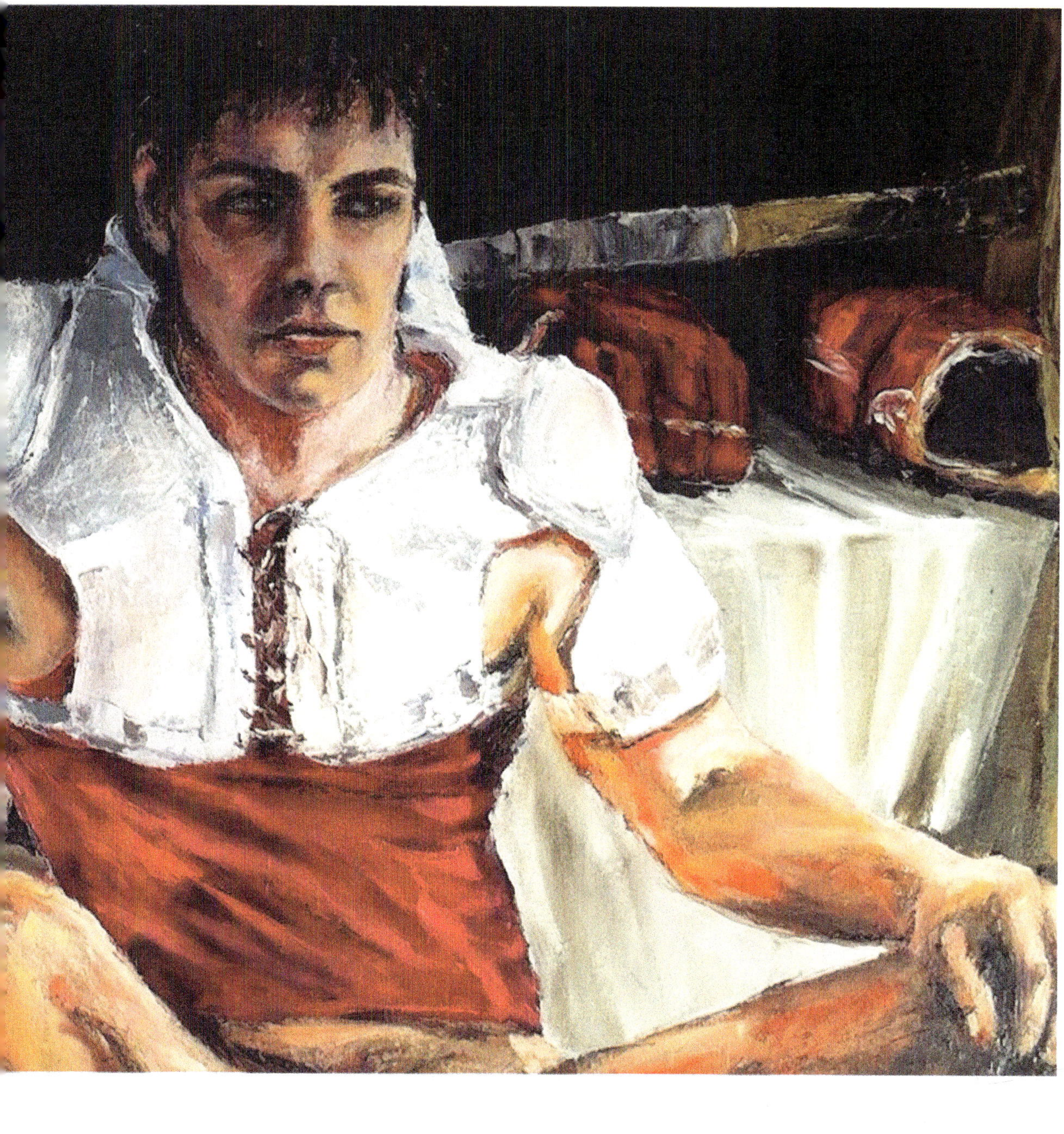

Ethica Press is an independent publisher exploring the interstices between gender and sexuality with a particular focus on queer and sex-positive non-fiction.

Ethica Press
Toronto | Vancouver
ethica@ethicapress.com
www.ethicapress.com

"Silence and Threat" by Michael V. Smith is adapted from *My Body Is Yours* (2015) with permission of Arsenal Pulp Press.

"Barebacking" by Simon Sheppard is reprinted from *Sodomy!* (2010), with permission of the author.

Front cover image: "Zeitgeist" (detail, modified) by Pablo Cáceres.

Back cover image: "My Boyfriend Walt Whitman" (detail, modified) by Michael Horwitz.

We thank our friends who shared their own stories in ways that reflected and challenged us.

We are grateful to our partners, Mark, Bradford and Josh for their loving support on this journey.

For his invaluable contributions and commitment to this project, John E. Brennan.

For their keen eye and years of inspiration, thank you Ed Wolf and Michael Anhorn.

For those who have spent their lives in service to our LGBTQ communities, including our mentors, you are the inspiration for this journal. Thank you for the freedoms we have today. You showed us that by claiming our worth and living out loud with authenticity, society will evolve with us.

Marcus Greatheart
Robert Birch
Pan

CONTENTS

Foreplay

Robert Birch
Marcus Greatheart
Pan

What started as a conversation between friends in the hours just before New Year's Eve 2014 grew into a hardcore inspiration. Three friends came together to wrestle with the belief that the expression of gay men's sexuality has shifted in light of advances in HIV treatment in recent years. We knew it to be true and had stories to share — our own and those of our intimates — but what wasn't clear was how to pull them all together. None of us had a lot of time: Robert is a doctoral student working on a PhD in the social dimensions of health for gay men, while Marcus is finishing medical school with an interest in LGBTQ health, and Pan is an artist and elementary school teacher. Initially we thought we would simply photocopy a few stories and images and bind them in some aesthetically pleasing way. But as the submissions arrived we realized this work needed to be shared more extensively. So we reached across our networks and into the interwebs, asking folks to share their reflections and experiences on the topic of an HIV zeitgeist for gay men — and this anthology is the result.

We brought our own unique editorial perspective to this process. We are social educators, health practitioners and artists operating for 20 years within gay cis/trans men's communities in the Pacific Northwest. We are queer feminists who share similar investment in the importance of how stories impact our community. As editors we intentionally play with an ambiguous 'we' throughout this introduction in an attempt to rectify silences by giving voice to our shared lived experience within community. We advocate that what happens to some of us, affects many of us. We are white, university educated and live with a great deal of privilege, which we attempt to mobilize here by sharing these important issues for the benefit of our communities. This book represents the culmination of a 18-month endeavour for which we take responsibility and also feel sincerely blessed. These are our truths and we hope the narratives printed here will help ignite dialogue and art among our readers and communities.

Between these covers

The premise of this first volume of *Annals of Gay Sexuality* (AGS) is this: we've entered a new era of gay men's health as it relates to HIV in terms of identity and practice. This shift reflects gay generational differences in terms of how we relate to sex, risk and community, advancements in HIV treatment and AIDS care, and the obvious: decades have passed since AIDS overwhelmed the gay male psyche. This journal responds to the belief that we're chronically overdue for our collective psychosomatic check-up. Our method has been to gather stories and images as practice-based evidence with the understanding that:

a) creative expression can be healing;

b) art has the potential to rekindle community efforts to organize around gay men's contemporary health crises; and

c) understanding more about the lives of gay men and the sexual contexts within which we live, our efforts will lift us out of the decades-long statistical impasse of HIV prevalence by addressing gay men's health as a whole.

To this end we adopted a unique community-based methodology wherein we sent out a Call for text/image contributions, and selected the work we believed best demonstrated how gay men are navigating their sex lives today. We are the curators of these submissions using a community centric lens. The text and images selected both express and discover the vigor and limitations of the editors' community networks. By contributing to a larger conversation of gay men's needs, this project seeks to expand into other culturally specific and global networks. At the end of this introduction we reflect on the work included among these pages.

We intend to stimulate conversations amongst gay men. We chose print as the medium because we understand the respect the printed page garners among the people and institutions we hope to inform and influence. May these ideas invade libraries and break down walls in academia and health authorities while challenging assimilationist norms within our own communities. *AGS* borrows from the milieu of health science journals that fill academic libraries. By appropriating this medium, we hope to challenge and entice traditional researchers and institutional(ized) practitioners. We invite those who judiciously map out what we do to embrace the expression of those who are doing it. In this journal, experience narratives create the knowledge that quantitative data and meta-analysis often overlook.

The title of this journal, *Annals of Gay Sexuality,* is our way of stating that we want to explore the visceral edge between what we know and the biocultural outcomes we still seek as gay male writers, visual artists and lovers. 'Annals' comes from the Latin 'annus' meaning a year, and represents our desire to capture emerging issues of gay men's sexuality.

The Contemporary HIV Zeitgeist reflects our intention to encapsulate present-day tastes, textures, sights and smells of our sex in the context of current HIV treatments, but also the social contexts of the fourth decade of AIDS. The text and images are immediately raw and thoughtful, erotic and cogent. They include personal narratives, photos, 'txt msg' conversations, social media posts, and non-fiction poetry and prose. This explicitly subjective work is experiential and defiant, self-reflective and critical.

AGS includes visual source material about the body, desire, medication and fantasies that cue up responses to the multitudes of present-day gay male sexuality. The theme among these images is clear: how artists negotiate with—and manage their relationship between—the body and sex. For some it was the fractal patterns of the capsules and tablets that allow gay men to live; for others, it's a fictional relationship with dead poets, reimagining one's youthful body tumbling through a fantasy of desire and intimacy. Some of these artworks are more explicit, arousing and demonstrating the higher potential of the body: sex and its many beautiful and messy complications. Other works resist the explicit.

We find it ironic and a reflection of our time that some artists are still unable to be explicit in their expression of gay male desire, despite increased political liberation. Case in point: the *AGS* Art Director was not comfortable using his legal name in this publication because, as a licensed public employee and educator, he feared that a colleague or student's parent might bring his propriety into question. Gay men who work with children are always subject to greater scrutiny than our heterosexual counterparts. While only two other contributors requested a pseudonym, the issue of privacy is one with which many of us grappled. We have public and professional jobs that provide us a lot of exposure. And while we were not convinced that our participation in this project would necessarily lead to overt discrimination or loss of employment, the potential risks still felt palpable.

Cultural health is an ally to personal health

We need each other now as much as ever. Thank you AIDS Inc. for the meds but clearly they're not enough. Pharmaceuticals will never replace the need for chosen family. While the pills protect us and keep us alive, close friends and quality lovers guarantee our quality of life. This is not ingratitude; this is a renewed call for help. As a population, gay men are in a state of despair.[1] Since 2007 our rates of suicide

1 The US CDC cites that as of 2013, 75% of reported primary and secondary syphilis cases are among guys who have sex with guys. www.cdc.gov/std/syphilis/stdfact-msm-syphilis.htm

replaced HIV/AIDS as our leading cause of death.[2] Crystal meth use and syphilis also demand our immediate attention. Our numbers in terms of anxiety, depression, suicidality, self-harm, and other mental health challenges are significantly higher than heterosexuals.[3] We need help, and many existing services often fail us. Mainstream healthcare models created for heterosexuals don't work for many gay men no matter how much we pretend they do. Many AIDS service organizations do not have the capacity to meet our needs today. We desperately need queer/trans healthcare reforms. Our healthcare processes depend on cultural frameworks that help us understand our bodies, our explorations into gender and sexualities, and our histories, as well as our inherent homo-value within our chosen responsibilities to community. Helping others means helping ourselves. We need to relearn how to become each other's most effective allies.

Our needed queer skills

Trauma irrevocably marks us. Not one of us as gay men, whatever our age, has made it through this epidemic unscathed. We're all transgenerational trauma survivors of AIDS and homophobia. HIV will continue to be associated with gay sexuality for decades. We're

---

2 In 2007, suicide surpassed HIV as a leading cause of premature mortality for gay and bisexual men. Travis Salway Hottes, Olivier Ferlatte & Dionne Gesink (2014): Suicide and HIV as leading causes of death among gay and bisexual men: a comparison of estimated mortality and published research, Critical Public Health. See also: Haas, A. P., Eliason, M., Mays, V. M., Mathy, R. M., Cochran, S. D., D'Augelli, A. R., ... Clayton, P. J. (2011). Suicide and Suicide Risk in Lesbian, Gay, Bisexual, and Transgender Populations: Review and Recommendations. *Journal of Homosexuality*, 58(1), 10–51.

3 As one of many examples: Przedworski, Julia M. et al. (2015): A Comparison of the Mental Health and Well-Being of Sexual Minority and Heterosexual First-Year Medical Students: A Report From the Medical Student CHANGE Study. Journal of the Association of American Medical Colleges.

also aware that relentless homophobia often negatively impacts the acute political and medical support needed for others including women, Indigenous people and people with AIDS in the non-Western world. As many of us in North America delve into our generational histories we experience a multifaceted resistance to, and acceptance of, survivor's guilt. We screwed our way through multiple losses, isolation and sex panic to discover we're still here. Our sex lives flesh out our need for, and act as our tools of, change.

While trauma can debilitate it can also, willingly or not, cast us into new roles as cultural change agents. Coming out as queer/trans is a political act that can be devastating. It can also, with the support of community, be a health-promoting, culture-evolving offering. Finding each other and sharing our scars and strategies can be exhilarating. Healing from trauma requires survivors be seen as valued individuals, witnessed (when ready) for their nightmare, honored for their survival skills and celebrated as vital members of community. By kicking the closet doors open, by bravely being ourselves, our sociocultural initiatory practice compels us to embody the role of culture brokers to the betterment of society. Coming out develops and demands a profound set of intrapersonal skills such as courage, strategy and psychosocial adaptation. It is an imperative that we research the skills that queer and trans folks develop and deploy in shifting their social standing by coming out. Looking beyond coming out solely as a process could prove to be revolutionary. It's in our blood.

Our collective story is extraordinary. We must remind ourselves where we've come from if we're to fully comprehend the potential of what we can create. Many of us lived and died for sex. Over three hundred thousand gay men in the USA died of AIDS during one of the most profoundly loving human rights movements in history.[4] We

4 www.cdc.gov/hiv/statistics/basics/ataglance.html

have yet to lovingly claim the victory of our dead brothers against a near biocultural genocide. As with survivors of other wars, only those extraordinary men and women who lived through the AIDS years can fully comprehend the horror of those times or know the depth of love that gay men and our allies shared. If we are to find joy in our own wellness we must choose to remember them, be ever curious, and uphold and celebrate their extraordinary contributions to our lives and indeed, the world.

If we see ourselves as seminal to evolution rather than a biological aberration, our storyline gets far more interesting. In only four and half decades we've run the proverbial gauntlet. From invisibility to disco ball frenzy, near annihilation to killing ourselves with meth to learning how to find intimacy with transmen — all the while participating in the world where everyone else is also working out their shit.

Imagining Stonewall as our LGBT cultural birthday, it is no wonder we are in the throes of a full-blown cultural midlife opportunity: We are 46. While we gain mainstream rights, we need to learn how to reorganize in real-time communities. We may shirk our social responsibilities in favor of re-exploring the erotic-cultural adolescence we missed. We may be shtupping our way into a full-blown queer cultural renaissance. As we queerly mature, let's envision ourselves as the loving Daddies we never had. We also need intergenerational mentorship to entice our mental, emotional, physical and spiritual wellness. For this to occur we have much more compassion slinging to do.

Greater and more imaginative political actions will once again serve as a method to promote our overall queer health. Whether we choose it or not, our sex lives are political odysseys that can be used against us, or help us build healthier futures. We know the psychosomatic and social costs of stigma and hatred.[5] Many of us have remarkable tales of survival. Our methods of adaptation are the template needed for LGTBQ community education and health. Together, we are the change we seek. If we click our heels three times and say, "There's no place like community," we might recognize each other as miracles-in-waiting. When we see ourselves as members of a diverse community invested in the culture of queer/trans* health — not just as gay men focused on HIV — we envision rewriting the HIV narrative with the overall intention of improving our lives, inclusive of the sexual health of future LGBTQ people.

Where in the risk are we?

There's a paradoxical (n)e(u)rotic movement emerging amongst gay men. How we hurt ourselves may in turn be how we learn to heal ourselves. We assert that sexual choices need to be appreciated before being 'understood' or 'influenced'. To begin to understand our deviance from any idealized norm, we look to the patterns of change affecting our lives. The convergence of our histories with biomedical advances, the hyper-prevalence of technological communication, and global crises characterize these capricious times and greatly impacts our erotic abstractions. We've been rewriting the sexual risk narrative.

Over the past year we've noticed that the gay guys we know, love, and fuck, are having sex differently, particularly in how they relate to/with/away from HIV. We observed multiple discords and envies between poz and neg men within our communities. New epidemiologically inspired identities, their accompanying politics

5 As of 2003 homophobia costs Canadian taxpayers 8 billion dollars annually. www.usask.ca/cuisr/sites/default/files/BanksHumanCostFINAL.pdf

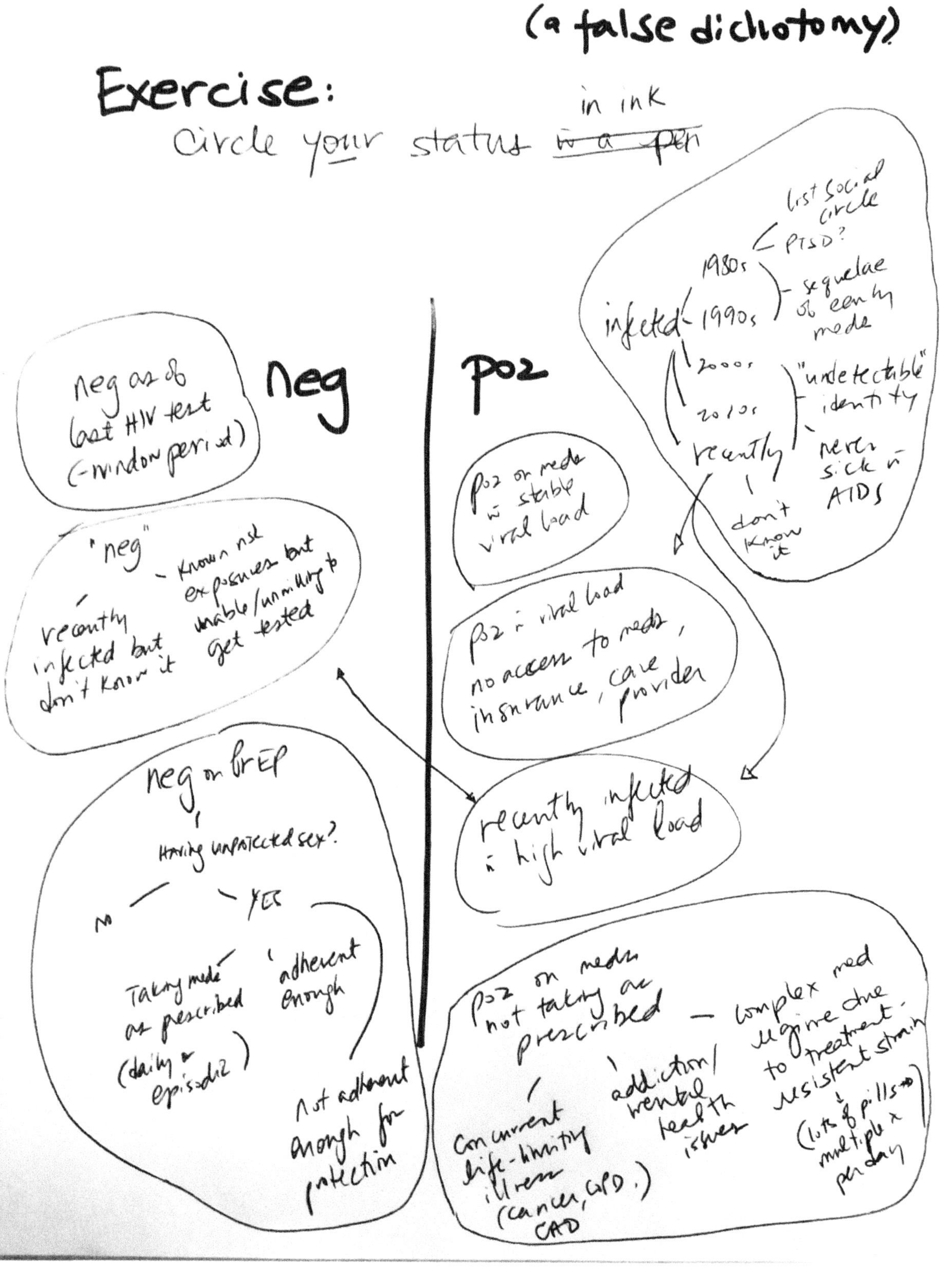
(a false dichotomy)
Exercise:
circle your status ~~in a pen~~ in ink
neg
poz
neg as of last HIV test (-window period)
"neg"
recently infected but don't know it
known risk exposures but unable/unwilling to get tested
neg on PrEP
Having unprotected sex?
no
yes
Taking meds as prescribed (daily or episodic)
adherent enough
Not adherent enough for protection
infected
1980s
1990s
2000s
2010s
recently
lost social circle
PTSD?
sequelae of early meds
"undetectable" identity
never sick w AIDS
don't know it
poz on meds w stable viral load
poz w viral load no access to meds, insurance, care provider
recently infected w high viral load
poz on meds not taking as prescribed
concurrent life-limiting illness (cancer, COPD, CAD)
addiction/ mental health issues
complex med regime due to treatment-resistant strain
(lots of pills multiple x per day)

and viral hierarchies have surfaced online within gay circles.[6] In light of emerging research on Antiretroviral Therapies (ARVs), Pre- and Post-Exposure Prophylaxis (PrEP/PEP), and Treatment as Prevention (TasP), we recognized some guys adopting new risk-benefit analyses for sex without condoms.

What we first poetically imagined as a sensual ripeness in the air amongst our friends and lovers is now strutting across gay male sex scenes toward a new sexual (r)evolution. What proof do we have of this? We, as gay men, are finally talking about ourselves again. We wear 'Truvada Whore' t-shirts and participate in online bitch sessions about PrEP. We're discussing the release of the Partner Study[7] which suggests 'undetectable' may mean it's not only safe to bareback a poz person on meds with no viral load, but it may also be safer (statistically speaking) than sex with a negative guy who doesn't have an up-to-the-last-shag HIV test. Despite real concerns about STIs, many gay men appear to be practicing "all rubbers off."

Always progressive in the realms of technology, we faggots lead emerging intimacies and technological ecstasies. We flirt with online geographic proximities, choosing to 'share my location' on smartphone hookup apps to scout out potential trysts, and where many of our poz buddies are using (+) as a shorthand for self-disclosure. At the same time, 'transgressive turn-ons' that are too dangerous for the real world become virtual beat off material with rare consequences. We embrace slut shame and attend group sex parties as if they were neighbourhood potlucks. As we transgress, so we progress.

---

6 As far as virtual communities go, consider the potency of the Facebook group *PrEP Facts: Rethinking HIV Prevention and Sex* which has 5,822 members as of March 14, 2015, agitating for the uptake of PrEP against an understandable resistance to sex without condoms.

7 Download the report at: www.cphiv.dk/portals/0/files/croi_2014_partner_qa.pdf

Sex = Health

Sex generates many biological and social benefits, stress reduction not the least of these. Sex gets us out of our heads, into our bodies and helps us live for and in the moment. Sex can be a spiritual high. Peak sexual experiences help us temporarily transcend a world bent on (our) self-destruction. Sex helps sweat out the chronic state of homo-hate many of us experience. On a good night, the sliding on and into each other's bodies can be tremendously affirming, validating in many kinky ways. We can appreciate many of the 'self-destructive tendencies' that cannot be captured in the 'stages of change' and which no public health messaging is going to deter. We need sex- and substance-positive community health models ready to catch and/or cheer us on as we stretch beyond our hard comforts. We know isolation is the killer. Those of us who benefit from the resources of the industrialized world—as consumers of pharmaceutical and users of technological privilege—have a responsibility to be of service to those who have yet to make it out of our well-lubricated black holes.[8] Much more needs to be shared about the healing benefits of sharing our stories. The contributors in this journal graciously dish out their own rough-and-tumble-out-of-bed episodes, revealing more of what is happening in these liminal erotic spaces.

Building a case for our (sexual) stories

Such narratives invite empathy and imagination. As we learn to tell our gloriously messy stories our way, perhaps we'll see enough versions of ourselves to experience greater relief from our present day

---

8 For a way to learn skills of how to talk about the complexity of sexual negotiation and disclosure see: www.hivequal.org/hiv-equal-online/the-secrets-of-learning-to-master-de-bate and for the radicals amongst us: www.reactup.fr/ and www.facebook.com/ThePinkPanthersMovementThePinkPanthersMovement

stressors and recognize that we're not as isolated as our silent grief and fear would tell us. To evolve we must be witnessed for coming through vulnerable and painful times of change. HIV epidemiology has been brilliant at laying out the groundwork for our understanding of how gay men have been impacted by HIV. However, we cannot expect clinical research to tell the whole of our story for us. Our HIV statistics are certainly not as stimulating as some of the tell-alls gathered in this journal. A colleague recently said, "If I was to live my life by statistics alone, I wouldn't ever do much of anything." We argue that our stories will inspire needed (re)action more than HIV statistics can alone. Re-storying ourselves will flesh out these numbers. We're counting on it.

Since the advent of AIDS we've heard gay men accuse researchers of following the agenda of the pharmaceutical gravy train in pursuit of their own careers and at the cost of community programming; that we've been left to fend for ourselves as they work on their mathematical models and abstracts no one really reads. The truth is that great work has been done and translating these findings to our diverse communities has been tepid at best. It's seems to have taken a full generation of prevention workers to get their Master's degree to understand and begin to act on these findings. Our stories augment decades of HIV/AIDS statistics and the significant body of work by MSM researchers. Our lives have been described by MSM theories in terms of minority stress, resiliency and syndemics.[9] We encourage people new to these concepts to learn about them and spread them

---

9 Minority stress (e.g. homophobia), resiliency (a strength-based individual and cultural reframe highlighting our hard work of bouncing back from the epidemic) and syndemics (describes as an aggregate of two or more diseases within a population under stress from multiple health disparities such as poverty and structural violence that in turn make us more susceptible to the burden of disease).

into the queer commons. We have many fierce researchers and allies working on our behalf.[10]

REFLECTIONS ON SUBMISSIONS

We are editors and contributors, and held ourselves to the same ethos that we requested of others. We wrote about us, not them, preferring to take responsibility rather than lay blame. By participating in this inaugural journal we agreed to erect/enrich/eroticize the conversations we've been privately indulging in, now envisioning this as a community-culture making process.

Who has time for faggot shame anymore? Reading **Joshua Barton's** *Slaughter the Moonlight* and his biblically proportioned sound bites makes my lustful heart lurch in disgust. This hyper-indulgent dystopian slop-house revelry makes me want to claw at my crotch and jack off in my own blood before smoking a pack of cigarettes then casually light myself on fire. It reminds me of a brilliant young fago-lala I met two summers ago, suicidal and gratefully too talented to do anything about it, when we talked queer his only response was, "Burn it all down, the parades, the rainbow flag, the basement bars, all of it." He would find a soul-mutant in Barton. I re-read the piece a month later, loved it, and then took a blister-raising shower. [RB]

Because we're different, gay folks possess a freedom the moral majority both denies and craves. **Francisco Ibáñez-Carrasco** describes how pain and envy shaped him as a young sissy boy during the torment of the 1973 Chilean *coup d'état*. *Can You Hear the Drums Fernando?* delves into the healing paradox of BDSM culture where

---

10 *AGS* wants to give a shout out to the decades of work by community and clinical researchers especially through the annual B.C. and Ontario Gay Men's Health Summits.

the writer reveals how he transformed boyhood torture through chosen erotic subjugation. The author's sexual quest for emancipation travels through four revelatory decades of politics, pop culture and AIDS to arrive at our current biomedical machine, the Pharma-domination of our still undefeated queer community. His story is a profound act of faggot self-determination. By harnessing pain in order to harvest pleasure, Ibáñez-Carrasco nurses his own suffering world-view and so invites the reader to consider how they too may have turned their misery into some life-affirming kink. [RB]

RM Vaughan sets his group sex essay, *Scheune House Rules*, in a dilapidated Berlin bar before acknowledging the demise of the gay scene. Even gloved sex has devolved to the status of 'retro.' He inquires, "How is asking to use a condom a threat to someone's health status?" and challenges the cultural-controlling term of 'barebacking.' He asserts his self-determination to use a condom as a queer erotic revelation. In his post-scriptive imaginative pick up line he reminds us where we come from, that queer requires some make-believe, it means erotically making it up together as playmates of a shared dungeon [RB]

We live in an age of techno-desire. From our 'addiction' to porn to our endorphin bumping phone apps such as Grindr and Scruff, are we truly enjoying our high-speed sex lives? In **Navid Tabatabai's** poem, *Tonight*, following his own quest as a self-described 'sacred slut,' he dares us to re-imagine an online hook-up as an attempt to merge the spiritual within the sexual. He reaches into the anonymous void of our pixilated realities to more fully embody ecstatic man-on-man communion. [RB]

AGS Co-editor **Marcus Greatheart** (soon-to-be) MD is the dreamy kind of doctor for which many of us would gladly bend over and cough. Smart and sexy, he brings two decades of community street-savvy to the often panty-tight halls of Public Health. In his piece, *Please Come In: Early History of 'Bareback' Gay Pornography and the Internal Money Shot,* he fights from our corner to say gay men and other man-on-man porn lovers are more than capable of separating fantasy from reality. From the conviviality of 70's 'natural' porn onward he closely follows the cavity-investigating lens of gay pornographers and current film buff-loving analysts. Marcus takes the pulse of our 'bareback' fetish to hear the throb of us beating-off to what some think of as our birthright: skin on skin penetration. In his sassy trademark style, this finely written article positions articulate pornographers up against the pan-paranoia of gay sex moralists. While judiciously not taking sides he certainly writes the script for future check-ups. [RB]

What mainstreamers will never quite fathom is that when gay men gather, cultural shifts percolate. While the rest of us napped, hung over from our frivolities, **Mischief** and Marcus lounged on the guest room bed. In *See Dick Fuck* these two dear friends share their pillow talk. Our glitter-littered house was full of sissy boys and hairy cowgirls draped over the worn out furniture. Two things happened that weekend: this journal was conceived and a long buried conversation sprouted its way into these pages. It's inspiring to have quality friends whose gift of reflexivity opens the precarious door to lovingly dish about poz-envy and sero-negativity. What makes this conversation dangerous is that it is rarely spoken out loud. Wrapped in each other's arms these two friends, in and of itself telling of what our peoples need most, expose today's poz guy privileges and neg man burnouts; the beast in the room that haunts us all regardless of our viral status is stigma. This piece offers us a once 'undetectable' view of what is now possible across the HIV paradox that has so connected/ divided us: admiration for our stamina. [RB]

In *This Feels Good, Though,* poet **Timothy D. Rains'** primary images of blindfold, spider, teeth and rope are woven together into a lusty contemplation on risk that builds anticipation with his syncopated musicality. In *How Can You Be Beautiful To Me?*, he explores longing and desire for connection that, for many of us, is a dangerous temptation; it risks exposure, infection, and opening one's heart and being vulnerable. [MG]

Michael V. Smith, in a selection from his 2015 memoir *My Body Is Yours*, explores how both our first sense-of-self as a sexual being and our first sexual experiences replay and echo through our later sex lives. These ghosts help and hinder, and are particularly vibrant when HIV haunts the halls. The work is both sexy and insightful, demonstrating deep wisdom as he adds to, and simplifies from, within the complexity. [MG]

Robert Birch shares lurid and (autoethno)graphic data that inspired his PhD research into gay men's group sex environments. The fellow really throws himself into his work and subjects (with consent, of course) and the result is a narrative meditation that is equal parts porno and travelogue. We started calling him Dr. Orgy, the intrepid student traversing the seediest and sexiest parts of North America in search of queer truth and a good blowjob; he claims the name with pride. [MG]

Eric Sneathen describes his work *For Gaëtan Dugas* as a series of cut-up poems which bring together significant cultural texts on a topic and reassemble them with scissors and glue — in this case a (false) history of the beginning of AIDS embodied by the nominal French Canadian flight attendant. The general process for a cut-up is simple: take multiple printed documents, cut, tear, or rip them into pieces, and bring them back together with tape or some other kind of adhesive. Eric explains that he is "trying to build narrative that relates the polyglot experience of the bathhouses, what might be the quintessential queer locale of the pre-history of the crisis." The poems evoke a flurry of images, like the morning-after recollections of an intoxicated night at the baths spliced with flashes of men and their body parts. Today they seem to be sites in-between times, both before and after AIDS which, in our minds, is an important concept to consider on its own. The poems offer a new historical methodology that, in my mind, is as compelling in product as it is important in creation. [MG]

Is *Barebacking* a real life story or fiction? Is **Simon Sheppard** talking to himself or is he othering? The narrative voice suggests self-denial while simultaneously implicating the reader. Are we caught red-handed? The protagonist wants what he wants when he wants it, without accountability. And yet, he seeks amnesty in the discussion when challenging our ethical sluts. What are your politics around sex with a married man? Thanks for the dare, Simon. Discomforting enough to be compelling. [MG]

Our desire evolves into cultural phenomena. Using 'txt as image' we have **Wilson Copland's** *Steamy Boy Puss* in which he takes us on a self-lubricating ride with a hot trans/cis date with two tops vying for pleasure-holes. The piece offers a snap-shot of queer folks sexually working out profound gender-cultural differences using online app-speak to evolve our kink in ways we may never have imagined a few short years ago. [RB]

Our cover image, "Zeitgiest" by **Pablo Cáceres,** utilizes two common tropes within painting: the mythic and the portrait. His figure walks the line between innocence and ruin, a creature of agency and restrictions. [Pan]

Michael Horwitz's vital and fictional relationship with the author of *Leaves of Grass* depicted in My Boyfriend Walt Whitman is both intimate and humorous. There is great power and magic in the fantasy that Horwitz creates with the combination of text and image. I love most his sense of play between the fictional and the dark actual goings on of life. [Pan]

In "Clean/Dirty" and "It Adds Up," **Grahame Perry** deals in patterns, structures, and dichotomies, and yet they are all about survival, striking the line between being clean and dirty through everyday objects, to using fractalized patterns to negotiate the relationship between survival and dependence. [Pan]

"Time Out" from the series *Vulnerable and Exposed* from painter **Lore Schmidts** is perhaps the most realistic and simple of the journal's visual selection. It depicts a man in an idealized form, young, built, and in the rituals of sports, but my favorite part is how the evidence of the stroke of the brush helps us to realize that even these creatures are constructions of the artist. [Pan]

In **Wes Fanelli's** "Believe it or not, there was a time in my life when I didn't go around announcing I was a faggot," the points of entry into eroticism include men in suits eating and the communal act of devouring. The explicit act of eating gives way to an implicit sense of desire and community. The eyes closed are my favorite moment of simplicity in the frame. Fanelli completed a series of work similar to this piece, and each used his real life friends as models. I can't help but be reminded of Mapplethorpe's "Man in Polyester Suit" and how the excitement of sex and pleasure are hidden by the formalities of suits and ties. [Pan]

Childhood play is the focus in **Pan's** "Gothic" and "Touch." The work places a group of men as survivors in some wild landscape. Instead of focusing on survival, they find sustenance in the acts of childhood games: tag, picking flowers, and hide and go seek. In the depth of their play, there is a hidden eroticism yearning to come out at each moment of their touch.

*

We acknowledge there are many more voices needing to be heard, especially those of trans men, male immigrants, and men of color.

We reached out to our man loving networks in the English speaking, western world and these stories represents much of what arrived. We envision this journal as an opening to a more fluid/loving dialogue between cis/trans/gay/queer/bi male flavored artists, academics, activists and other down on your knees storytellers.

This is the first edition of *AGS*. In the next edition we plan to explore gay sexual ethics and amories (more about that at the back of the book). As the new ones on the journal block we intend to be incendiary, political, unapologetic and subversive; we embrace our necessary queer failures out loud. We hope to spark your imagination and interest and, in the spirit of healthy critique and community, your feedback is appreciated.

*

Join the conversation online at www.annalsofgaysexuality.com

Silence and Threat

Michael V. Smith

Silence and threat have been like smoke in the fabric of my sex, wafting in, finding seams and settling. They were there even in my first days of fooling around at age ten, with a boy who had 'evil' in his name. It was 1981. "Bette Davis Eyes" was the number one song by the smoky-throated Kim Carnes, Prince Charles married Lady Di, Nintendo introduced North America to their first version of Mario in Donkey Kong, and The Centers for Disease Control and Prevention in the U.S. announced that five gay men in L.A. had a rare pneumonia.

To mark the spirit of the times, let's call this boy Knievel, after the motorcycle daredevil, Evel Knievel, inducted into the Guinness Hall of Fame for "most broken bones in a lifetime". He was all over the TV in the early 80s, jumping over buses and shark tanks. For a birthday present that year I was given an Evel Knievel action figure, with a pull-cord powered motorcycle. I was a not-yet-queer kid: a stunt jumper in white leather was hot shit. He had no fear too great to challenge.

The Knievel in my class felt just as reckless. He was two years older than me, but only a grade ahead. He'd failed grade one or two. Sydney Street Public was a small school, so grades shared a room, three and four were together with Mrs. McClelland, while five and six had Mr. Thompson, the aging bachelor principal. I don't remember Knievel having any friends, partly because he transferred into the school late, in grade five, I think, and partly because he was a bad mix of aggression and unpredictability. In hindsight, I think he was more hyper than violent, but as a young fey kid, it was hard for me to discern the difference.

On the day for class photos, when we'd line up in the gymnasium shortest to tallest, I was in the first half, around the third way mark, usually standing behind Julie Legue and ahead of Jennifer Khalil. It was the 70s, so my hair was long and shaggy. My voice was alto. My eyelashes were thick brown butterfly wings. Often I was mistaken for a girl. It was a confusing time, where I failed often at decoding what was appropriate for "boy", so when Knievel's busy eye settled on me one day—he invited me over after school—I swallowed my fear and said yes.

These were the months in my family leading up to my parents' first separation. My father would return from work on payday Thursday, drunk, much too late for supper and with little of the paycheque left, to find the door deadbolted. Because my father was alcoholic and my mother was a screaming hysteric in response, I had learned well to compartmentalize, to slide in opaque walls around what happened at the kitchen table that morning so I wouldn't have to look at it for the rest of the day, or ever. A lot of my childhood landscape was like a shipyard of storage containers, the days stacked and invisible, one row against another. This was our normal. Silence and threat.

In our quiet aftermaths, I'd lay in bed imagining ways to escape, sometimes jumping out the second storey window, or using my Star Wars sheets to lower myself down. Sometimes I'd slip to my death, sometimes I'd jump on purpose, head first. Sometimes I would drop onto the roof of the car and run across the road to live in the tall grasses in the open field across from our house. Sometimes I'd hitchhike or walk all the way to my grandparents' house, an hour's drive away, and they'd take me in. They'd hide me. Or I'd run down the steps and out the front door, into traffic. I'd time it for when a transport was passing, to be thorough. I lived a great deal of my early childhood feeling like I was alone at the bottom of a deep well, shouting upwards, with nobody bothering to peer over the lip and help.

When Knievel invited me home, I felt like he'd thrown down a rope.

He lived with his maternal grandparents in a corner house just a block and a half away. When I knocked, he opened the door seconds later, with a girl standing just behind him. He introduced me to Lee, his sister, whom I wasn't expecting. Lee had a 70s cut of brown hair that lay straight to her shoulders. Her bangs dangled in her eyes, the same kaleidoscopic blue as her brother's, but without the wildness.

The two of them had had their last name changed to match their grandparents, after they'd moved in. I remember being told by someone, vaguely, that they'd had trouble with their parents so they'd been taken away. Because their grandfather worked at the paper mill, the household was financially comfortable. They had a nice bungalow in a neighbourhood that was mostly small wartime houses, built in the 1920s. By comparison, a 50s bungalow made them well off.

Knievel and Lee brought me downstairs—I didn't meet their grandparents on that first visit—to play a game of hide and seek in the unfinished basement, with the lights off. We abandoned that when I couldn't bear the blackness. Their alternative was to play another game, in a fort Knievel had built along a wall in the basement. I'm not sure what it rested on, but the fort was a few feet off the ground and enclosed by walls on all sides. A wooden door slid back revealing a carpeted space about the length and depth of a closet, but only 3 feet high or so. Just tall enough for us to sit with a small clearance above our heads. There was a desk lamp in a corner that Knievel turned on. All three of us piled in, and Knievel slid the door closed.

For this second game Knievel and his sister said we were to take off our clothes. When I resisted, Knievel looked me in the eye and said calmly, "I won't be your friend unless you do."

Most everything about that moment has stuck with me these thirty years, the ultimatum, my stomach turning with nerves, the intensity of his blue eyes, his quiet, clear tone of voice which said this was true, I could be cut out so easily.

With our clothes off, we took turns directing a mix and match of body parts. Michael puts his nose in Lee's belly button, her arm on his leg, a foot on a bum. Knievel and I took turns paired with Lee. It was equitable, in that we did rounds of choosing, so that Lee had her turn picking who and what. We stayed loyal to the gender mix, strict boy and girl. As we went round, the dares grew more intimate or bizarre. Long hair dangled in a butt crack, lips on an ear, finger in a mouth.

We played this an hour or more, until I had to be home for supper. I don't remember much of the time in between, though I've a clear sense of my nerves. I was sick to my stomach with fear for what we'd done. Never had I had such a secret from my parents. I was accustomed to keeping private our lives at home, monstrous with fights. But my parents were accomplices. This secret was mine, and Knievel's, and Lee's, and nobody else's. Here was the beginning of a great privacy from my parents.

The second time we played this game, Knievel and I were alone. I knew what to expect this time, so the thrill of the experience was lessened, until I suggested the pairing of body parts that made Knievel uncomfortable. For me, our measure of success was how much it could make our stomachs flip and flutter. If it didn't churn our insides, it wasn't worth doing. I'm not sure what, but I suspect Knievel had something else in mind; he was more timid with me alone. He didn't like the tables being turned, where I was comfortable, pressing forward beyond him. At one point, he insisted we stop, but my curiosity wasn't done. I pulled out the best threat I had. "I'll tell your grandmother," I said.

When Knievel agreed to continue, I felt a rush of heat run down my arms and legs. We positioned ourselves in more combinations, with Knievel resisting every other suggestion. We had a push and pull on each one, some I managed to talk him into, others he flat out refused. In hindsight, it was all pretty innocent, given that neither of us were sporting erections yet. We stopped about the same time I ran up against my own level of discomfort. We had exhausted the body parts I felt drawn to pairing—I wasn't yet interested in anything penetrative—so we reached a point where there was no need to continue. I left that day with an odd sense of trembling in my body, a kind of wave. The knowledge that I had managed to humble the wild Knievel worked on my psyche like a low electric current. I had possessed a power to change a boy's behaviour.

A week or so later, Knievel chased me around my back yard, despite my yelling at him to stop. He was too loose with my body that afternoon, around other people, running after me, tackling, picking me up. Partly because he knew what we had done (he could expose me, we could be found out) and partly because he was too wound up to be aware of how people perceived him, Knievel was dangerous. Careless.

As he pursued me around our swing-set, I threw a seat behind me, smashing him in the chest. My mother saw us, and because my fear of being caught by my parents outweighed my interest in continuing the game, that incident put an end to hanging out. I ignored Knievel's invitations after that.

I have carried this dark sexual mystery—bodies that whisper, in uncertain, potentially threatening circumstances, playing with power, trading a sort of shared secrecy, aware of the strangeness of another, the strangeness of intimacy—into the most charged sexual moments in my adult life. Being with Knievel is how I learned to be vulnerable, to give in, opening my hand and releasing caution, trusting the heat of the moment will be greater than the risk. The kiss I gave my first boyfriend in the back seat of his mother's Malibu when we were still virgins began in that same silence, that hush of uncertainty, pushing shame and a fear of the unknown aside to release the heat running circles in my loins. It was there when I slipped my mouth around his dick the first time. The hush followed me, or I followed it, hunting that intensity which doesn't show itself when you speak too loudly, or too much.

For the six years after I broke up with that first boyfriend (we were together from seventeen to twenty-one, with gorgeous years of sex in there) I was more than satisfied swapping blowjobs with random hook ups, or occasional butt sex with condoms. Then in 1998, like a cheesy gay movie, my buddy Brad shepherded me to San Francisco. He was a nurse, a decade older than me, who had lived on the West Coast some twenty years more than me. He knew things. We stayed at Beck's Motor Lodge, on Market Street, which he brought me to as an awakening—the three-storey motel was notorious as a Castro cruising spot.

Every guest was male, except one wife in a Midwestern couple who may have known they were in San Fran but didn't know the exactness of where they were. Many of the other guests left their doors ajar and sat on the bed, hands strategically placed on their laps, watching a slow trickle of men pass by. Throughout the weekend, a number of guys at different times stood in the doorway to their suite, wearing a small white towel, or less.

Within minutes of arriving, Brad and I passed our neighbour on the walkway. James was likely in his early 40s, a thick mustache, half a foot shorter than me but easily with fifty pounds more muscle on him. He had the look of a good vintage porn star, with sweet blue-collar manners. In denim. He was famous in California, he said, for being the first out homo police officer, though I can't remember for which city. After meeting him that first day, I was brushing my teeth in the bathroom when I heard the shower start up on the other side of the wall. My knees practically buckled at the thought of him lathering his body.

After two more small chitchats, James invited me to his room to 'hang out'. Though I couldn't believe my good luck, I was super insecure, so considered not going. Brad was jealous enough that he wouldn't let me turn down the offer. "You just walk next door and knock. That's all you have to do," he coached. "The rest takes care of itself."

He was right. I knocked, James answered, and he invited me in. Fag life can be that easy.

Through a series of odd steps where I didn't quite understand what all was happening, James orchestrated a white towel on the bed, both of us naked, me lying on my belly, he on top with his large hard dick slicked up and pressed at the button of my ass. He was trying to wiggle his thick meat in my butt, bare.

I asked him over my shoulder if he wanted a condom. I had some in my jeans pocket, on the floor by the wall. I had only ever barebacked with my monogamous first boyfriend; it's easier to stay HIV-negative if you're really good at (and really into) blowjobs.

James whispered in my ear, "We're only cuddling, Mikey. We're just going to cuddle." But still he played his dick at the entrance of my butt, pressing and wiggling, until the head was definitely stretching my ring of muscle. That's a sensation you never mistake, especially with a dick as thick as his.

We played that loop a few times, where I asked for a condom and he shushed me insisting we were just cuddling, wiggling his hips ever so closer, until the fur of his pubes met the fur of my ass. He was buried to the base, breathing in my ear how much he liked cuddling me. There was so much repetition of that breathy language I was sure he was playing out some old history. I was a lucky geek filling in (being filled in) a part of a story he felt compelled to re-enact.

The edgy heat in my gut from barebacking had me cum within seconds. And he, clearly disappointed in me, pulled out. Let's skip the rest, where he popped sleeping pills and for the next hour I tried to seduce him while he slept or pretended to sleep. As with most one-night-stands, the denouement was anti-climactic.

For a good dozen years after that incident, I could replay the cop's hot breathy voice while I jerked off saying those words, *We're just cuddling*, and cum in a heartbeat. I cultivated that memory, I planted it in the soiled loins of my psyche. The cuddling cop carried all of the best qualities of a great sexual moment for a gay man. Most of us who lived our early years in the closet—with the threat of AIDS in news reports, all those deaths and protests—knew the silence James was rocking us towards.

In the park after the sun has set, as the moon drops diamonds of white-blue light through the tree cover, few of the men are speaking. They wade through the dark with gestures, responding to a touch with another of their own. For those men who choose to date first, then fuck, the bedrooms of gay dating aren't much different.

Silence is an echo. A paradigm.

We came of age not speaking. The hush was there before we began to shave, in our confusingly clear dreams, watching the knuckles and biceps of our friends' dads, in the sleepovers of temptation, tackled on the playground and jostled on the bumpy school bus. We learned what was hot in secrecy, so that, as easy as smoke, secrecy seeped into the fabric of that desire. Secrecy is no longer just a useful veil in how we do this or that, but it's become the thing we desire. We prefer to slip on the worn old clothing of silence to get lucky.

When you approach silence, and its cousin, fear, they open like automatic doors onto Sexual Thrill.

I've given or taken a dick in either hole with more than a couple thousand men. I think. I stopped counting when I reached around 1500. It's all hubris after that. In the last ten years, most of these men barebacked. Or tried to. Seventy-five percent, maybe? Seventy-five percent, I'd hazard, have tried to stick it in me, or to get it slipped in them, without protection. They say they don't want it, but when you get them alone in a quiet spot and someone's cock is in the crack of someone's ass, they nearly always forget their best intentions. I've had enough sex to know with some confidence that my ass and dick are appealing for a wide range of men, but I'm not so disillusioned as to believe I'm anywhere near the kind of god that would be worth risking HIV to have me raw for a half hour. So the high rate of men who want it bare isn't about how hot I am.

The men were met in bars, public parks, beaches, bathrooms, peep shows, porn theatres, sex clubs, bathhouses, and a wide collection of homes, including mine, in many cities in North America and a modest few in Europe. If we weren't cruising in public, we met via social media, via chat-based websites or apps, which is a new private kind of public. And I've been dating before Grindr, before Gay.com, before backrooms disappeared from most of the gay clubs. I might not be a social scientist, but I've had enough exposure with gay and not-so-straight casual sex to feel confident in my ability to say a few things about sex amongst men who aren't friends or partners.

Everything we don't say in the privacy of our sex lives creates room for thrill. Thrill of walking a line of sexual danger, thrill of being caught, or found out, thrill of being able to project onto that clean white slate who I want them to be. I am often in a sexual moment trying to find the edge of a desire that is verboten, where neither of us dare speak aloud in the dark, working us into a complicity of risk. If I'm not doing that work, the other guy is. Equal measures. Knievel introduced me to that dynamic as a child, James reinforced it in adulthood.

All the teaching and shaming and common sense and knowing better of HIV-prevention are no match for my need to be wanted, to use sex as a short-term filler, or fixer, for a gay kid raised to think he was less than. We fuck for any number of reasons. We keep secrets for any number of excuses. We fear any number of fears. Our silence and the threats we fear predate all sexual acts.

But during the sexual height of being penetrated without a condom, I have no perspective on the consequences of that behaviour. If the sexual alchemy is correct, I transcend the silence, I conquer the fear. With a raw dick in my ass, there is no tomorrow. I am at the zenith of intensity, which is a kind of darkness without memory, and, so, the intensity knows nothing of regret.

Here is another echo. The heart-racing fear I sought out in my early days is what I seek still, only the stakes have needed raising. I'm not saying that my past with Knievel, or a California cop, have caused my sexual history, that I have been determined by this and this and so here is the end result. We are taught to be victims of our narratives; we believe a past event makes us the people we are today. Some of that is sometimes true.

I want to propose our futures can just as easily determine our past—the things we longed for in our first fumbled moments of sexual awakening and practice are those that we fumble towards in our adult lives. What I sought with Knievel is the same needy, make-me-feel-worthy quality that brought a cop's raw dick in my ass. And a few dozen after him. It is not the past that might see me gracefully contract HIV and beyond, but a sense of being empty-handed, looking forward, without company. That longing—because it is an unanswerable need—will always be the future. It will always have consequences.

I remind myself that my actions at this moment in the present are most likely to determine the next. I'd like to inscribe in my blood the knowledge that all decisions are now; now is a perpetual moment of change. My past is finite and cannot alter, so why have I fooled myself for so long to believe that what has happened to me then will necessarily determine what happens next? Raised in a fucked-up family, spending years in the closet, I clung to the promise of tomorrow, that the future would be better than today. But now is always better than the unattainable.

It's so obvious it seems idiotic: secrecy needs fear, fear easily bedmates with secrecy, both are a lure for sexual longing in gay men, a fleshy carrot walking us to the precipice of safety. Speaking does or doesn't happen in the now. Barebacking happens in the now. Contracting a virus or being cautious against it happens in these moments, now. And now. And now.

Over Page:

Gothic | Pan

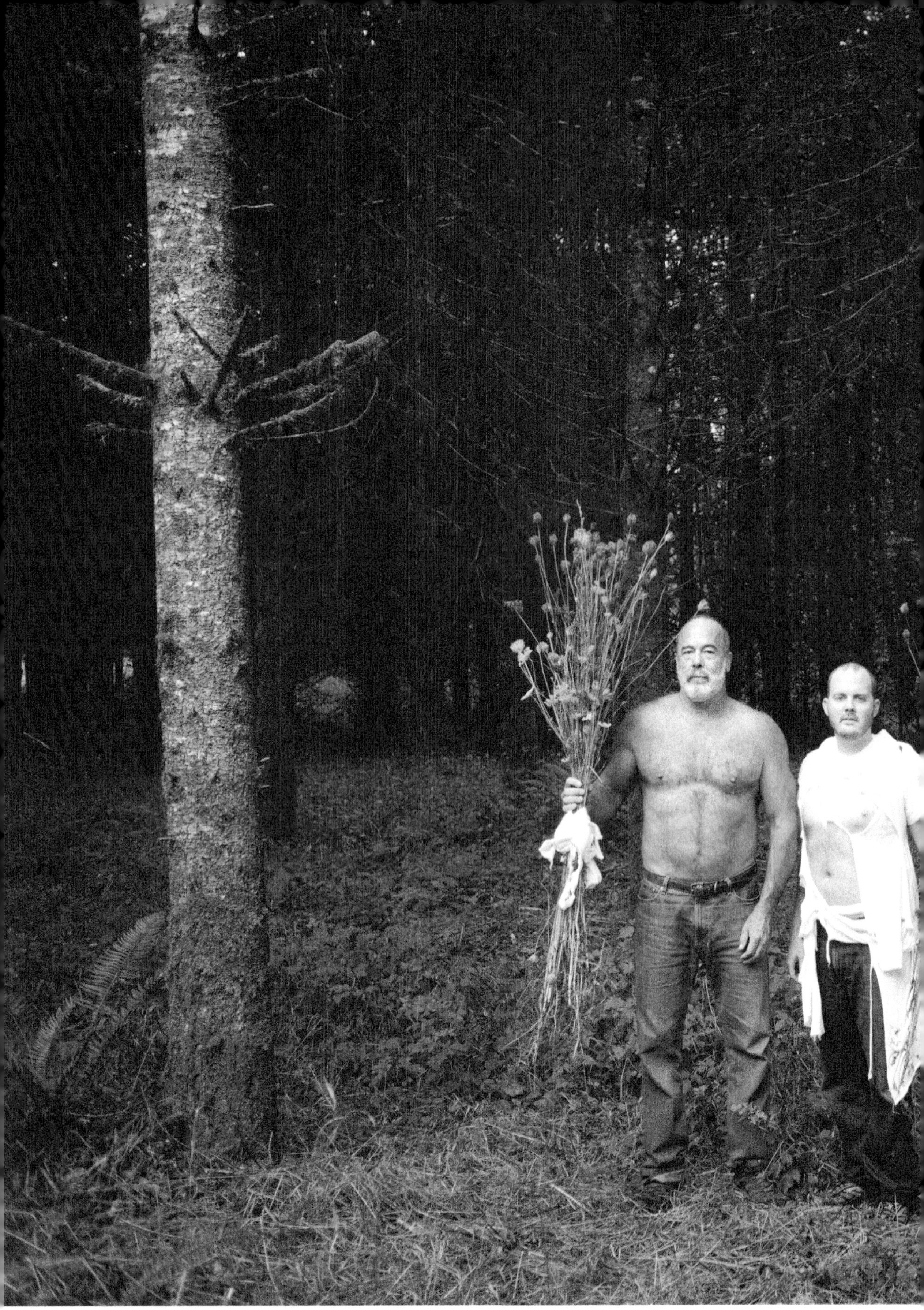

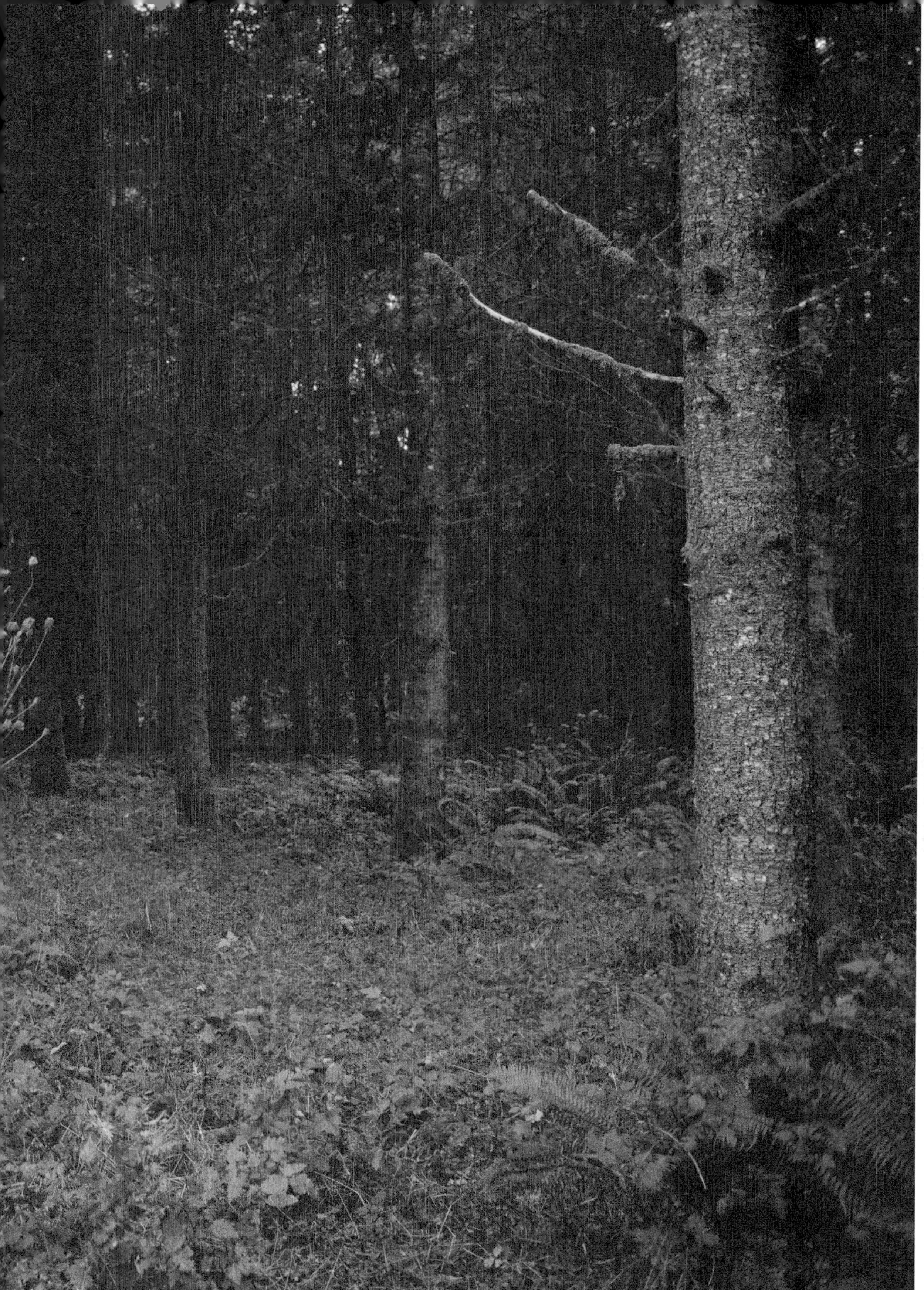

This Feels Good, Though

Timothy D. Rains

there is a black rope,
I carry between my teeth,
when I blindfold,
the spider crawling between my legs,
this feels good though,
you feel good though,
on the black rope,
carried between my teeth,
when I blindfold,
you the spider crawling,
between my legs,
you feel good, though,
I feel good, though,
on the black rope,
you carry between your teeth,
when you blindfold,
this spider crawling,
between your legs,
to feel good, though,
to feel this good, though,
I need to feel this good, though,
I need to feel this,
black rope,
crawling between my legs,
the spider carried between my teeth,
the blindfold feeling good,
as a black rope,
crawling between my legs,
a spider carried between my teeth,
a blindfold feeling good,
feeling good,
between the legs,
between the teeth,
between the legs,
between the teeth,
the spider,
crawls,
up,
the,
black rope,
blindfolded.

My Boyfriend Walt Whitman

Michael Horwitz

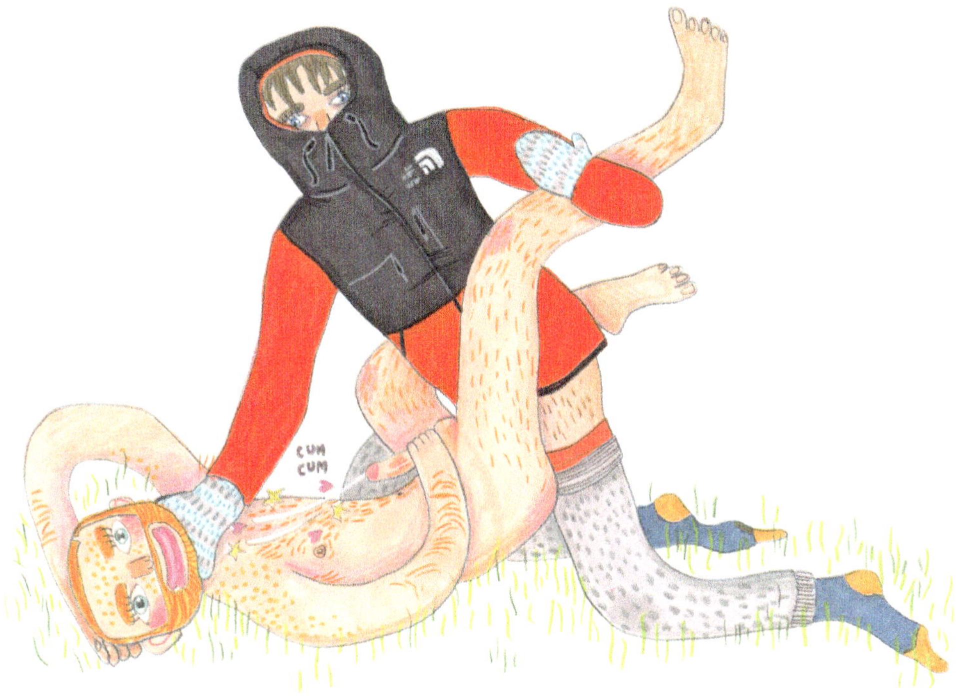

My boyfriend Walt Whitman is a poet who writes about nature and grass stuff and he loves to go camping and because I'm his boyfriend I have to go camping with him. But like I'm not a big camping person because I'm allergic to grass and whenever Walt is surrounded by grass he gets really horny and wants to bottom which is rare because he's like "I would never bottom" but he will if there's grass involved. he'll be all like "PLLLLEEEAAAASEE," so I have to fuck Walt in the grass and he cums as the grass blades go CRUNCH CRUNCH under his back and he is at one with the world. But since I'm allergic to grass I have to use protection and I wear two pairs of long underwear to make sure I don't get a rash.

Scheune House Rules

Fucking with the safety culture backlash in Berlin's darkrooms.

RM Vaughan

Scheune (English translation: Barn) is an old-school, "men only" gay bar located in the heart of Berlin's fading Gay Village, on Motzstrasse. Dark, smoky, beer and piss stained, Scheune is a relic from the 1980s and looks the part—old Tom of Finland posters, brown leather pummel horses/sex benches, urinals with two-way glass in front of them, a frisky, near pension age staff, disco, always disco, and, of course, old televisions playing old pornography. You have to be buzzed in. And that's just the first floor.

Beneath the bar is a labyrinth, a pitch dark maze. It has never been cleaned, or so I like to imagine. There's a sling (also never cleaned), a system of half walls and fucking corners, a spanking bench, a slave cage with a leash bolted to the floor (in the spot where there used to be a full sized bathtub-cum-urinal—how I hate change) and broken bottles on the floors. There are no monitors, no Dungeon Den Mothers, no supervision. One wonders if the workers ever go down there at all. It is a delightful free-for- all.

The only thing I have not done down in the grotto is have unprotected sex. And that makes me, I have learned from experience, something more retro than the very bar itself.

*

You can't miss the stickers. White squares with a thick black line drawing of an erect cock. The cock is ... how to put it? ... un-encumbered by latex. A raw cock. Over the cock sits a bright red circle with a diagonal line across it. You get it: No Barebacking. There is sometimes German text at the bottom of the stickers, but I read little German. The stickers are on the walls, on the toilet tanks, on the pillars, and on the rail that leads you down the winding, wholly un-safe, mismatched stairs that take you to the darkroom.

And then, they disappear, literally and figuratively, as if to say, "You can't say we didn't warn you", or "Due diligence, served." Yet, in the hundreds of times I have been to Scheune and sucked, fucked, and SM played in Scheune, I've rarely, and I do mean very rarely, seen any of my fellow enthusiasts using a condom.

But I insist on condoms, because I like to be fucked up the ass and not think, to empty my mind. A condom helps. A condom makes the man fucking me even more anonymous; he's just a dick and a body and a bit of plastic. I find condoms erotic. I don't expect other people to, however, so I ask that they be applied. The result? I don't get ass fucked very often at Scheune.

*

Look, I'm not a rules person. Quite the opposite. The only thing interesting to me about rules is how and why people break them, ignore them, or circumvent them.

In Berlin darkroom culture (yes, it is a culture), there are rules and there are not rules -- by which I mean far more than "the rules are flexible".

Here's how it unfolds: everyone knows that Safer Sex is the anticipated norm (and has been for a very long time), a now-naturalized power structure under which public health officialdom (some gay-run, many not) informs gay men that it is best advised that they use condoms during anal sex; everyone knows this norm, supports this norm (I have never seen a Safer Sex warning removed, peeled off, or scribbled over in any of the many darkrooms I've visited), and, when asked, will donate cash to initiatives to further this norm; and yet, as I have witnessed, approximately 10 percent of the users of Berlin's darkrooms actually practice Safer Sex—if anything, most men, when asked to practice Safer Sex, consider the request a challenge, indeed an insult, to their personal health status, cleanliness, and even sexuality/sexual prowess/masculinity.

How did we get here?

*

I dislike the term "barebacking", of course because of its idiotic cowboy connotations, but primarily because it reduces a complex system of sexual/power/body parts/body fluids exchanges to a *single moment*, the moment in which a condom is slid (or not) over a cock. "Bare backing" simply does not accommodate for the varieties of pleasures possible in condom-free sex, nor for how those pleasures can be negotiated within (or without) the realm of "safety". The term reduces a world of cultural and psychological issues to a single act, a penetrative moment—when in reality, negotiating one's own idea of sexual safety (or dismissing entirely the pervasive pressures of what can be a nanny-ish safety culture) involves the assertion/dismissal of a series of (often unspoken) sexual contracts, of moments, fleeting as these contract-establishing moments may be.

However, if barebacking (I'll use the term for—admittedly hated—shorthand here) is now the norm, not the outsider act, especially within the confines of darkened and anonymous spaces. Or, to look at it another way, perhaps gay men who use darkroom spaces have naturalized (and thus made quicker and more precise) the practice (and negotiating) of condom-free sex to the point where the shorthand term is merely a password, a nod and a wink.

Thus, we must consider, and challenge, how this popular (and popularized) term has been given so much power -- how it has grown from a term attached to a taboo to a pick up line, and how those of us who are the proverbial odd men out can try to reclaim a space within dark room culture that does not read our decision to use condoms (or, in my case, delight in the tactility of condoms) as un-masculine (the number of times I have told I am a "pussy" for insisting on condoms is too high to count), as conformist, as submissive to heteronormative dominion, as less-than-queer, as out-dated, as fussy, as prissy.

*

There is great power in the act of refusal. You have to give up some instant gratification (and don't get me wrong, I live on that particular drug), but a deeper power, one that lingers, comes with refusing to play by the rules. Or the rules that deny the first set of rules. Or, rules about rules about rules ... all of it, any of it. Just refuse.

I will not resign my power to ask for what I want. I want ass fucking with a thin layer of latex between my anus and whoever's penis. That's what I like.

If I accept that Berlin's darkroom culture allows for, and actively supports, a constant state of instability, especially in matters pertaining to officialized Safer Sex "best practices", then, by its very nature, Berlin's darkroom culture also permits me, must permit me, to function, and fuck-tion, in a manner that pleases me.

My decision to enjoy bum-fucking with condoms is as valid as anyone else's (allegedly rebellious, but now really little more than status quo) condom-free pleasure seeking. And yet, as a condom user, I have felt judged, dismissed, and de-sexualized. The irony does not escape me.

*

I keep a sex diary. Try it. Try it for a year. You'll surprise yourself after.

February 23, 2013, Scheune

Small crowd. Maybe 2 early? 11pm or so. Klaus, 50 (or just past/before), 6 feet 1, TV anchorman hair, TV anchorman handsome. Farm worker gear fetishist. Told me his boots were from a farm, a friend with a farm. Told me he gets trades boots with his pal every couple of weeks, wants the cow shit smell on his gum boots. Overalls and a thick tool belt. Rough. Went downstairs. 2 guys joined in. Fingering (me getting) and blowing (everybody to everybody).

Bend-over time, Klaus wants raw. Klaus narrates a fantasy of sex in a hut on a farm.

Me: I don't like raw. Klaus: take it. Me: I don't like it. Klaus: good farmboys do what the farmer says. Me: No.

Klaus goes, I suck off some other guy. Home early.

Imaginary landscapes, costumes, mind-play, roles. And still, a script ...

Meet me in the middle, handsome. I'll play some games you like; you play some games I like. We're queer. We're meant to be malleable, full of holes.

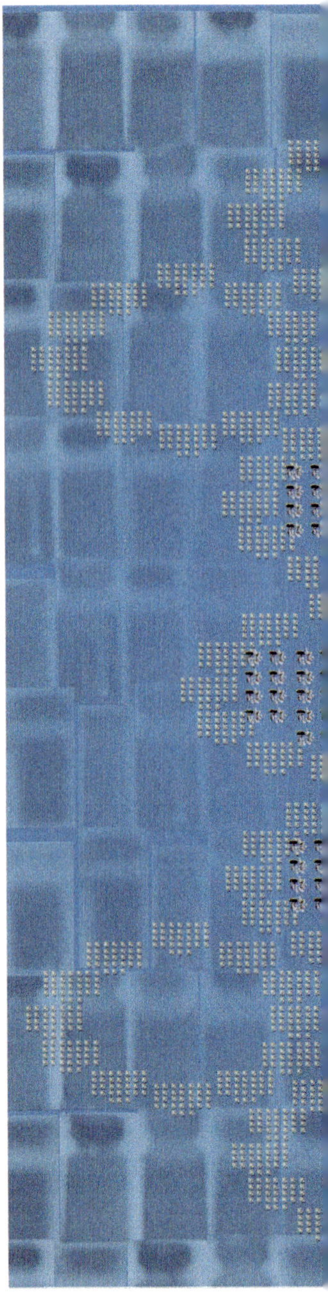

It Adds Up |

Grahame Perry

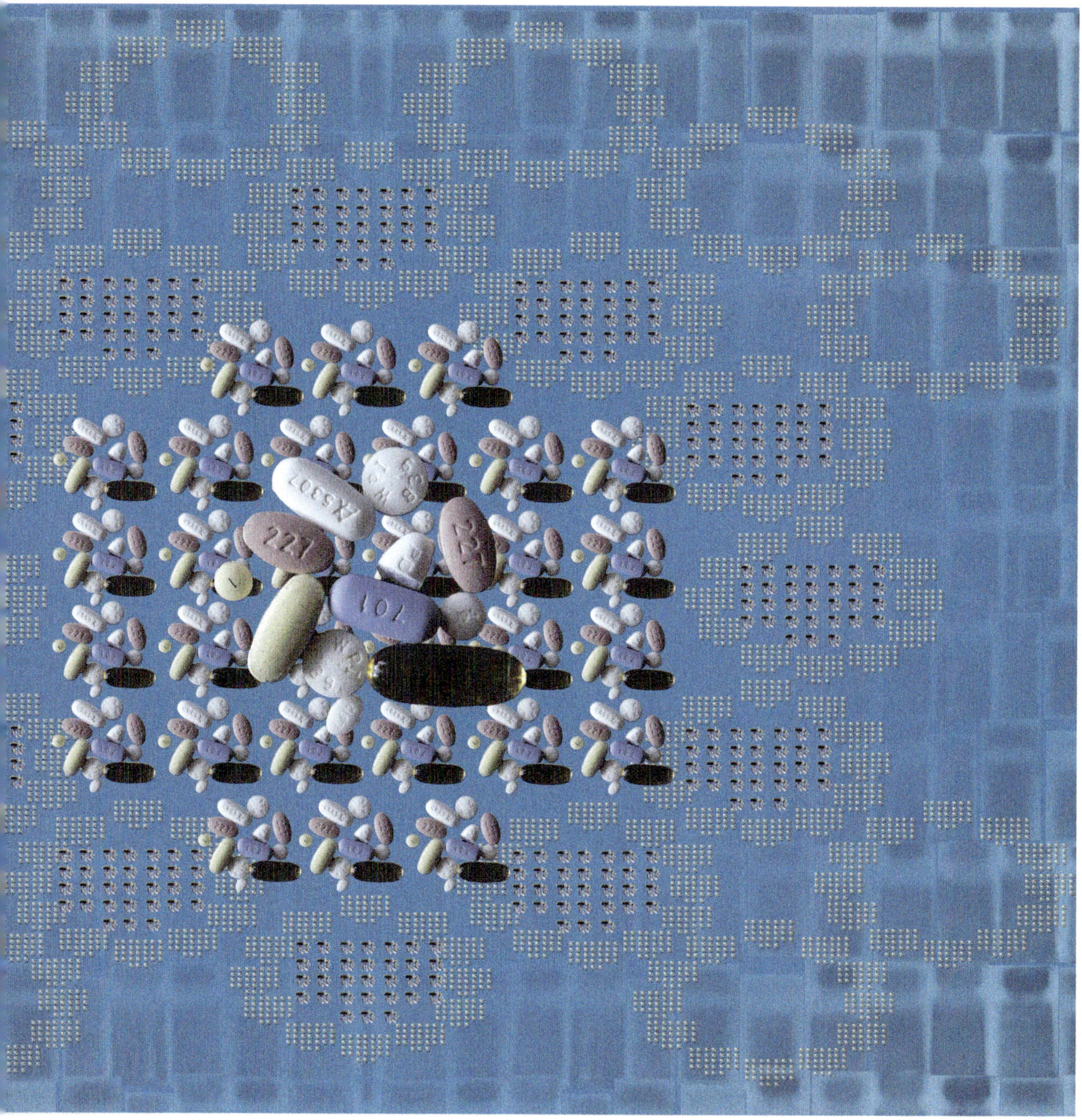

Slaughter the Moonlight

Joshua Barton

What are these moments of Paradise we find ourselves chained to when white nectars are released from the mouths of throbbing monsters? When our balls tighten and the warm blood fills our heads with shades of purple lusts, sweet syrups, the American dream drenched in poison cum and yellow piss.

American manhood is one continual hunt for meat and warm holes. Men are sentences running on streets paved with lies and nothing else matters but spreading their virus to a multitude of bare feet. Orange money shines through glass walls, reflects in pools of whisky on a wooden bar as Koko Taylor and Otis scream the blues. POZ pariahs message their midnight cruises with texts of blue orgy. They arrive at suburban sex parties like prophets on the hill in faded denim and hooded jackets. The bottoms work at inflating swollen purple balloons with their toothless mouths while grizzly daddies choke their cocks in leather rings. Tiny bottles of assorted nitrates litter the floor as a slobbering mass of men crowd around a doped up faggot on a semen stained mattress. The men penetrate the brown queer's pulsating hole with prize-winning zucchini, champagne bottles, crucifix dildos, pink canine cocks dripping with neon-green cum. There is no hope for humanity. The genocides keep a comin' like a slaughter of moonlight in the red nest of American superiority. Islamic boys eat ass to disco riots and burn Lady Gaga in effigy. More American bodies return home to Southern Baptist burial grounds and roach infested morgues...faggot throats are swollen rotten in Aleppo behind rubble dumpsters...the alleys are occupied just like the genitals...WESTERN minds are filtered with vintage colors...wars are re-blogged in the name of a free democracy, bluegrass songs, consumer-curated propaganda for god & country. The virus arrived in Gomorrah last winter. Word had it that pharma lobbyists had it engineered in the bellies of Sodom swine and sent over with those goddamn angels. It starts with a fever, vertigo, and a dull pain in the joints. She felt like a vicious dog. Always snarlin' and snappin' like a bitch in heat. American paranoia was now a communicable disease. 28 dead just two tweets ago. Hundreds of thousands bombed just two wars ago. Commercials for erections interrupt news footage of homosexual chariots in the streets of Canaan...Butchqueens make their asses clap for MERCY with sweet, tobacco stained skin....Golden glass pipes are loaded with Tom Ford nug as pungent vapors roll across peach lips and white porcelain like the ganja dreams of Kush children. Fat balls hang heavy with cosmic cum. Engorged, black bull cocks spit salty milk inside faggot jaws. Our minds hide in online temples of live sex ads, webcam porn, shopping cart iconography. We held the truth that we were all dependent on venom and viruses. Our amphetamine addiction was a warm fleece blanket from home. The ghost was gone and she left all her shit on the floor.

You wake up faded inside the stomach of an Atlanta jail smelling of piss and cheap sanitizer. You're bathed in vodka sweat as you chew on a slice of baloney. Soggy, white bread gums the roof of your mouth. ¿Te habla espanol? says the poor Mexican bastard sitting next to you on a dirty vinyl bench. You close your eyes and pretend to sleep. You've spent the last ten hours in the detention center's processing room arrested for stumbling drunk up and down sidewalks in Ansley Park. American jails are 24-hour DMVs only with drunks and prostitutes. It's Faggot Pride, and you gain some sick lemming comfort in knowing that you count at least four black butchqueens, one stunt queen, a chubby white dyke and one femme queen with black tracks and a green shirt all locked up with you waiting for their bail to come through. The stunt queen has the highest bail out of every fucker here ($3,000), while the chubby dyke snores stone-drunk asleep on the female-only benches. The guards call the femme queen SIR, while a yellow-eyed bum stares at her tits. A uniformed giant calls your name, and you fall in line with two homeless drunks. The guard hands out stiff blankets that reek of stale vomit. He leads you three outside the processing room and into a steel elevator. You're instructed to walk along the wall as he leads you into the general population cells. Echoing laughter melts like sugar on the floor through shower steam. Naked inmates wash their dicks and asses, while the others are scattered among plastic tables playing cards or reading Korans. You are wearing a powder blue 70's disco shirt, suede wingtips, and blue socks printed with marijuana leaves. Should have wore sweat pants to the bar. You have no memory of the past six hours. Thank you vodka. The last brain cells from the night are printed with images of a crowded queer bar....drunk faggots and black lesbians....giant drag queens...pissing drunk in the bar's back patio alley...a blurry white man puts his hands down your pants and hands you more drinks...He takes you to his apartment, and somewhere in between, you wake up lost outside on the street....**BLACKNESS**....Two of the last photos you took on the now confiscated camera are a selfie in an apartment hallway mirror and another of red streaks of light at a crosswalk. Laminated signs are posted on the jail walls. They read in English and Spanish: ¡ACTIVIDAD SEXUAL EN ESTE FACILIDAD ES ILEGAL! SEXUAL ACTIVITY WITHIN THIS FACILITY IS ILLEGAL! You're still not sure what he did to you.

Reptilian-Republican demigods and theocrats convene in Florida to celebrate more dead niggers on television while drunk delegates rape prostitutes in flamingo motels down the row. A needle poked femme queen rambles to a bartender about The Shangri-Las and her latest trick. Chipped, red nails tap-tap with each sip she takes on her beer. She slurs:

— SO THERE WAS THIS TRANNY AND she was down the block sucking on strawberry popsicles when this Earth was born. Her favorite customers were them south side cops cause they'd always be the ones to pay her bail. She loved sucking off the security guards 'round back of the discount grocery store. Bitch even got a train ran on her for sum damn deli meat!

She lifts her head off a pine pillow and waits for the faggots to unbutton their flies. READY AND WAITING FOR MORNING CUM. Sissy faggot traces circles in her nude pumps across beige carpet... walks in snorted lines anticipating the next trick's arrival...already done swallowed two loads but she still thirsty for forgiveness...Sissy wobbles her ass in the dark and pretends she's the oracle whore possessed by cum drunk succubi, faggot holy ghosts, a bottle of malt liquor. Religion, she says to herself, was the true threat to global security and national mental health. It was the reason for mass graves, seared flesh, torn arteries, ash hills, the VI RUS. Sissy wears a yellow burqa and works down by the south city tracks that run across Chippewa. She lets the stockyard crew feel on her tits in abandoned factory lots. The Cubans smell of cigars and brandy. They stroke her synthetic black hair as they coo: 'CHUPAR BIEN PRECIOSO....ABRIR SU CULO PARA PAPI'. The Bosnians and Arabs prove much more blunt in their tactics preferring to breed the Sissy with bareback anal orgies. She closes her eyes and prays for deliverance as double penetration lifts her up into Rapture.

WORDS ARE MOMENTS IN THE IMAGINATION WHERE OUR BODIES ARE CHAINED TO BURNING STAKES LIKE FAGGOTS IN HEAVEN. It seems as if everyone is a goddamn writer now penning lists of life lessons learned from 90's television and Lindsay Lohan. I continue to follow the vintage method of combining copious amounts of liquor, narcotics and a steady stream of fresh semen. This random I fucked in West Memphis doesn't recognize my photos and hits me up on Grindr to tell me he wants to shoot his load on my face. I text him that he already has. We met when I was in Memphis to find out why Duanna Johnson was found on Hollywood Street with a bullet to the back of her head after filing a major civil rights lawsuit against the city's police department. Instead, I ended up drunk and fucking at least 10 different dudes within my week stay. It wasn't unusual at the time for me to suck off multiple men a day. One sad bastard fucked me in the basement of some office building where he worked as a lobby rent-a-cop. I parked my car in a lot behind his building and walked inside the front lobby where he sat behind a high, gray counter in a khaki uniform. We said hello. He stood up and motioned for me to follow him along a side hall through a basement door. We walked down and into an abandoned back room that I realized was once a dentist office. The brown vinyl exam chairs left bolted to the floor. I sucked his white country dick before I climbed on top of him and ride him bareback in the dentist's chair. He was number three.

The fuck who sends me a message tells me that he remembers that I fucked him good. I text him:

– I'd let you give me a face full of cum again.

– That would be hot. But mine comes with an additive these days.

– hiv?

– Yea. My ex's departing gift.

– When did you find out?

– I knew he was positive. We were trying to be careful but he nutted in my mouth a couple of times. One time it was so far back in my throat I had no choice to swallow it. He broke up with me three days later bc he was afraid I was going to catch it. Oops. Too late buddy.

– Isn't it really rare to get infected by oral sex? Had you gotten oral surgery?

– It's harder but not impossible. He was recently poz so he was very contagious.

I'm not sure I believe him, but I tell him that I hope he's doing okay.

– Thanks. I just want someone to fuck the hell out of me and leave me with a hole full of seed.

Universal subjugation through viral infections was the next logical step for the mind control industry. Who needs a department of propaganda when the virus already comes complete with its own RIGHT WING RNA. It was everywhere: hypodermic needles, flu vaccines, the water supply, Big Macs. Everyone had it, because the government had manufactured the bitch. As she spread across the nation, the virus became labeled: GOMORRAH-RELATED-IMMUNE-DEFICIENCY. Sodom's top health officials were dispatched to Gomorrah to isolate the virus and find a cure. Meanwhile, Queero-Phaggot terrorist cells begin cropping up along the Mississippi. The Feds begin tapping faggot cell phones and tailing militant drag queens to porno safe houses. The pigs can't vomit up enough evidence to bring federal treason charges, so they hire recovering narco addicts to infiltrate the revolutionaries and plant plastique explosives inside suitcases of wigs and black butt plugs.

WHAT IS LANGUAGE BUT A SERIES OF IMAGINED BLACK SAMBO FACES, RED HOLOCAUST ON FRUITED PLAINS, HIVES OF YELLA JACKETS, DADDIE IN DENIM AS HE CARRIES YOU HOME SWADDLED IN A PASTEL KNITTED BLANKET?

– We're just faggot children lost in them green woods.

Jesse says to me as she sucks on her thumb in drag prophecy. I ask her:

– Evr seen her beneaf moonlight?

– You always askin' me if I've seen her....Have you seen her in holler mist lit by foxfire... Have you seen her naked breasts baptized in the church creek? Now you askin' if I've seen her beneaf moonlight? What the hell?!

– Yes. You seen her in moonlight yet?

– No. Not yet. Not ever.

Jesse passes me a lit joint. I take a deep drag from it and the vapors escape my lungs in a series of guttural coughs. Our minds glow with violet lusts as telepathic static drains like blood into the sky. I press my lips against the face of cosmic galaxies and ask myself if corruption was the defining characteristic of this wretched planet. My body is raw as the walls crumble outside Jericho. I see nothing now but memories of that yellow sissy lost in pine woods. Her cock throbs inside church pews as she stares at plump crotches of bluegrass banjo pickers in tight denim jeans. She touches herself and sings along with the congregation:

> I SAW THE LIGHT, I SAW THE LIGHT. NO MORE DARKNESS, NO MORE NIGHT. NOW I'M SO HAPPY, NO SORROW IN SIGHT. PRAISE THE LORD, I SAW THE LIGHT.

A swarm of mice are nestin' out in the barn chew'n thru the wires and soiling winter crops. Black widows hatch in rotten hay bales on a worn dirt road. The boys out back behind the church swalloin' salty piss. Daddie's sick again with shingles, and Grandma tells me I need to get right with The Lord. Orgasm spreads like a virus through the fields resulting in an explosion of rats. Natural resources expire and the population plummets with coordinated starving and chemical warfare. Pillars of salt sparkle in black eyes as the rats gather to watch the fires cleanse faggot land. The blue reptiles rub their engorged red cocks against themselves and leave HIV nectar in the palm of my hand. His body was dissolved into the ether of literature. Technology and all her sisters were infected with it too. No healthcare so you gotta take your daddie to the VA. No healthcare so all we gots is these shitty meds. Plains are burnt with holy wind as Job crawls from the cellar. Poverty is an egg rotting in the sun while the drones and the wasps buzz above the trees. Blood drips like honey as mutilated Muslim children weep over severed heads courtesy of New American Liberalism. There was always a queerness here in eyes rubbed red and raw with white oak pollen. It was in our country-dyke mothers and molested fathers. Winter air cracks like cold rusted trailers and broken meth pipes. Blonde hair and black blood melts with charred plastic bottles. Them boys on the run to Arkansas while skinny women snort lines of Vicodin off buttercup bathroom sinks. The house was always being rented out by someone lost out on Highway 72: Alcoholic mechanics, single-mothers with meth cook boyfriends and smelly children, a family of scrap metal hoarders. Lips are full with pink flesh and stained with white lakes. Blunts are smoked before banjee boys remove throbbing cottonmouths from their jeans. Orgy woods are lit with emerald lights while torn'ado sirens wail like mothers from Genesis. Whippoorwills call queer souls up out of these frozen hollers and into glorious hells. Momma whisperin' to me that at The End she'll know me better than Jesus himself. The night is long, and I can still hear the kai-yotes cryin' fer a slaughtered moon.

Shipped From: [redacted] Pharmacy   Date: 08 Apr [redacted]   Page:

[redacted]

Packing slip for:

[redacted]

Check: R&B	PATIENT	QTY	DRUG	Rx#	FEE	COST
	[redacted]					
		60	Atazanavir Cap 300 mg	[redacted]		1,345.98
		60	Ritonavir TAB 100 mg	[redacted]		86.27
		60	Truvada Tab	[redacted]		1,633.14

TOTAL FEE:	$0.00
TOTAL DRUG COST:	$3,065.39
TOTAL COST:	$3,065.39
TOTAL ITEMS SHIPPED:	3

Please reorder BY PHONE ([redacted]) when there is [redacted] weeks supply left. If you are leaving a message on the answering machine, include the name of your pharmacy or clinic, the patient's name, medication required and remaining quantities. Please allow 1 - [redacted] weeks for delivery.

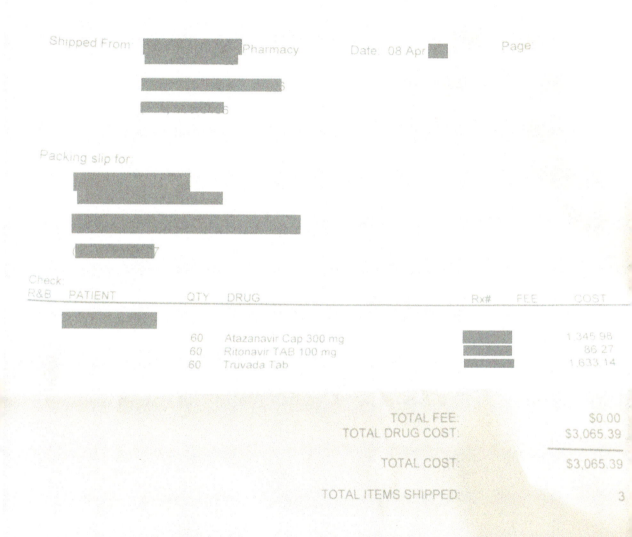

Tonight

Navid Tabatabai

Stomp, stomp, stomp:
Feet trudging up my stairs,
Bringing vibrations of possibility.
iPhone pixels have shaped destiny:
Sparked flesh into motion,
Desire pulsing through veins,
On his course now, up the doorstep,
Inside, he is alive - life itself, unstained!
But who is this man smelling of too much cologne?
This man at the beck and call of a phone?
This man selling himself with too few words?
This man saying, "I'm sorry, I've forgotten your name,"
And why bother remembering, he won't see me again,
This man who was denied Desire's kingdom
And is convinced now never to falter again?
Who is this man, Cosmic Mirror, but myself!

Tonight, we are fulfilling more than fantasy.
We are claiming more than the little pop-up box the world has granted.
Tonight we will be much vaster than "jock," "bear" or "twink."
Tonight we will join a tribe of fathomless esteem:
Great Alexander, forlorn Rumi,
Walt Whitman, David Bowie,
And those countless other sluts of ancestral glory:
Nameless - and shameless.

We start it, but it is more than that.
We call it sex, but it is more than that.
We are skin-on-skin holy communion,
We are diviners searching with fleshly rods,
We are nature uncontrolled, before civilization,
Following pleasure's heart with healthy abandon,

So that we can run off that cliff,
Of which orgasm is but a glimpse.

There is a call, response - stroke, moan - pinch, cry of delight.
We are here to dance with fluid and grace,
To trust the messages of pleasure and pain,
To stop crutching with guilt and dining with blame,
To give up the search for the man outside who'll fulfill us,
And to fuck this fleshly man who is alive and alone,
To find our inner man, the one with no name
And to grind it and squeeze it until we see they're the same.

But, in my heart — it's still scary to see you in the grips of passion,
Scary to see you awkward and exposed,
Scary to see you when you're dead and you're spent,
And my spit's in your hair, and your arm's on the floor,
Scary to see you overcome with nature,
Scary to see that this is the Truth.
Scary to see you never again,
Scary to see you as Everyone.

And after all, after all that was said and was done,
After all the awkward attempts at normal conversation,
After all the blood has risen and fallen,
After the cum has been shot and flung on the walls,
After all the laughter from contemplating the neighbour,
After all of it, all of it, there's a queer satisfaction,
To have tasted the feast offering, quivering, alive,
To be reminded again of the eternal orgasm.

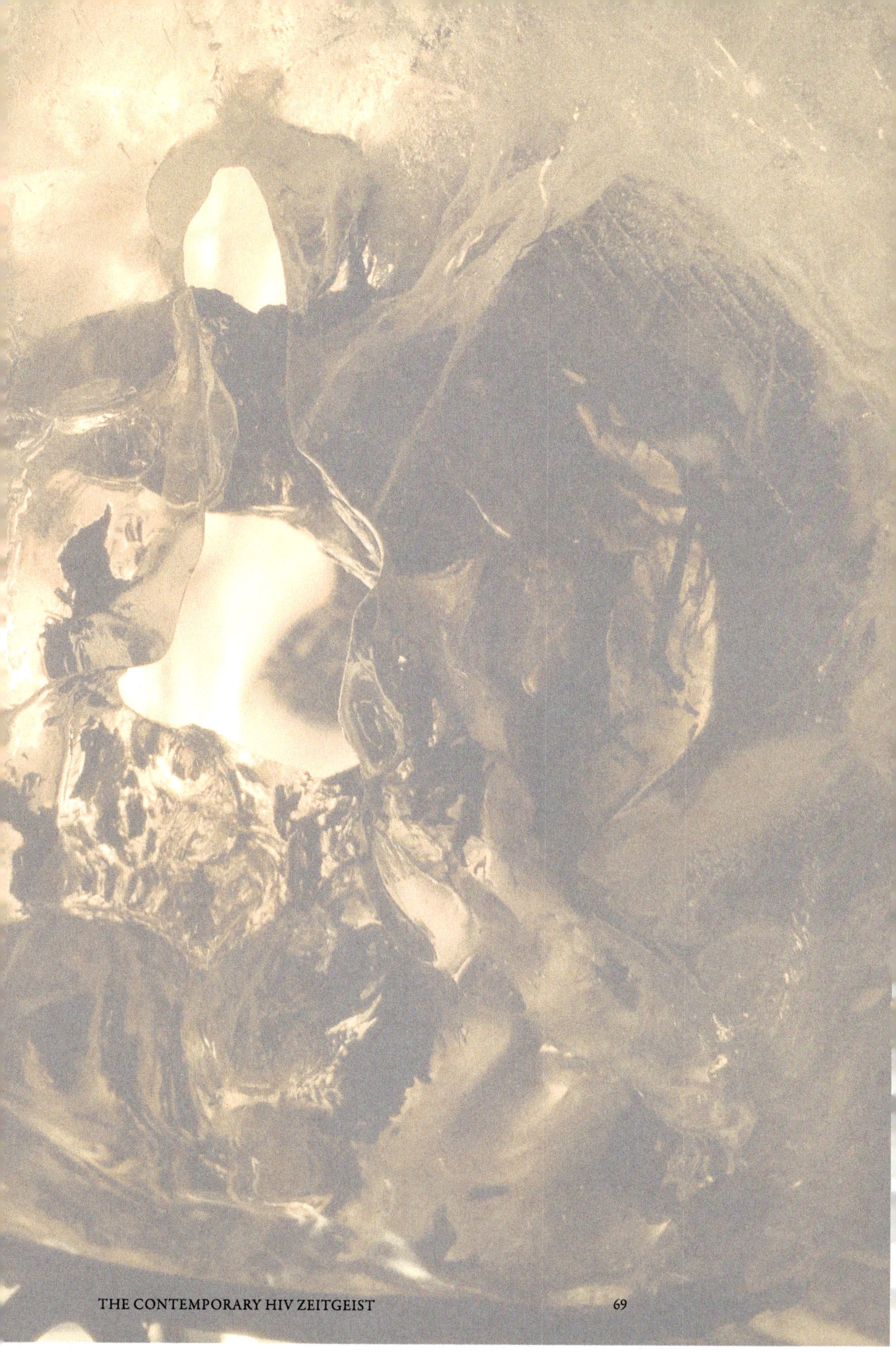

Right: Zeitgeist | Pablo Cáceres

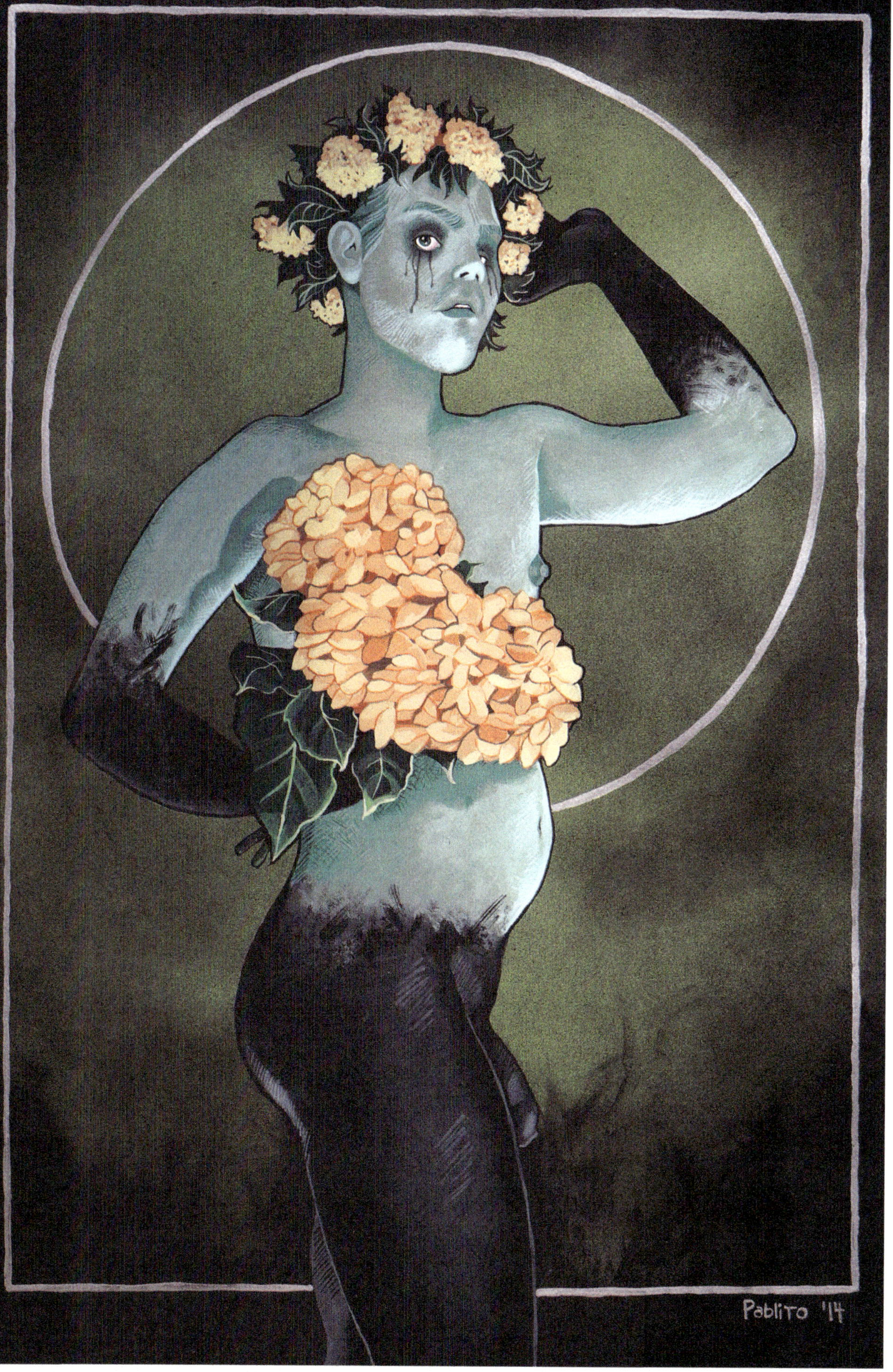
Pablito '14

Can you hear the drums Fernando? Or, my brief story of discovering pain and envy

Francisco Ibáñez-Carrasco

Pain and envy live in the gay erotic zeitgeist. In my life, pain is a necessary exploration; envy is the eyes that watch it critically. In the years following the Chilean *coup d'état* of 1973, recession and military dictatorship hit us hard. After years of living in uptown houses with manicured lawns, my mom Isabel took up a maid job in a household at the back shop of a floor tile factory in *Calle San Pablo* – the historic but dilapidated and rough *Barrio Matucana* with its long dark lines of 19th century adobe houses with double doors flat nosed up the sidewalks and no front yard was a far cry from the lavish modernity of *el barrio alto*. In the factory grounds burly dusty men would craft tiles from scratch, hours on end, sweating, and using a tile press. In 1976 I started high school at *Liceo de Aplicación* on 29 Ricardo Cummings Avenue. I was thirteen years old. The school was almost one hundred.

An old spinster employed my mom, a lovely fat Italian lady, *Señorita Carmen*, who over the years had taken in a motley crew of boarders, dogs, and this old factory inherited from her Italian family, a real albatross.

In that adobe house, right behind the front store where tiles were on display for sale, lived the old woman, and a young woman who was her protégé since her adolescence, and a nasty short woman with stringy hair dyed blonde, her own teen daughter, and her thirteen year old son, Fernando. In those times, in strident dissonance with our everyday reality, the ubiquitous radios turned on in every kitchen siphoned the angelic voices of ABBA intoning, "Can you hear the drums Fernando? I remember long ago another starry night like this..." Fernando was the first man to fuck me.

I was already in the habit of staying over time in the *Liceo* to avoid the grim reality that didn't fit my fledgling queer fantasies. Or I spent more time than any kid should in a dubious Teatro Colón at the corner of the Maipú and San Pablo St., a cine rotativo that showed three of four cheap movies one after the other all day, a three storey building that had seen a better past in the previous century. That's where I saw a damaged celluloid copy of *Cabaret*. At the Teatro Colón ticket booth, it didn't matter how old you were or what your intentions were. True motion picture experience.

In that household, my mom and I were given a small shack, a room with a wooden door, one bed, and a small window in the very back of the property, past the piles of new tiles, and the scary cement pools where the tiles were soaked once they have been made. There, I learned the price and function of my holes; I experienced humiliation and pain and liked it, albeit in guilt and shame. I didn't understand why.

Fernando had a membership to the YMCA which was a luxury to have at that time, and was sent to a private high school. He was masculine, outgoing, disdainful, and beautiful. He played skillful soccer and guitar, and swaggered with a smirk. I was bookish, shy, and effeminate. I only had school friends. Fernando's friends were mighty fine looking to me; they would come around in the afternoons to hang out. If I was around, sequestered in my shack at the back, reading, writing, they would come and taunt me, make remarks, laugh at my Farrah Fawcett poster ripped from a magazine, and push me around – that is how it all started.

All scientific explanations of why one child can get used to pain and humiliation, and then crave it, fall short of what I feel in the very fiber of my being. Shrinks and priests and elders and coaches and instructors have tried their hypotheses and remedies on me. I never wanted to be cured. I wanted to understand and explore. Pain and humiliation, by any names you need to give them to fit them comfortably in your world view, were an undertow and became a surge once I became HIV positive in 1986 and a hurricane after 1996.

Humiliation, the internal craving to be put down, submitted, subservient, or subjugated comes with being gay, the good sissy boy who does as told, no strut, no defiance. That child still lurks inside of me watching the micro-aggressions of others pile up. But there is a power exchange in every act, even that one of torture requires a certain sordid nurturing in order to bring the next lash to life. Every action of humiliation begs for the emotional physics of a reaction. It took time to become an invert and understand this reversal.

The boys in the *Barrio Matucana* came around checking themselves, showing off, and I guess my desire showed off in its own way too, wincing my eyes, batting my eyelashes, part resentment and part yearning and defiance. First, I was tense, rigid and hard, but a good altar boy, I swallowed every single slippery adolescent insult and serpent, every laughter, and every viscous expression down my pharynx. The way the priest who taught me to have sex with him before my adolescence said it should be, the way the church goes down, a potion of slippery violence, shame, and spirituality.

Are shame and guilt and hurt a singularly lonely prison or are they forces that can be redirected? Don't they call this "resilience"? How is it being down on your knees, filled and mocked, akin to being in control of yourself and the situation? Isn't the "bottom is always on top" a throwaway sentence? In the next forty years, I grappled with this somewhat cliché notion: *the one who loves you hurts you* (or flogs you), and understood it very distinct from *allowing oneself to be being constantly hurt,* offended, victimized, or thumbed down. One is the use of one's power differential in paradoxical and productive ways; the other is being swept away by the undertow of power. An interesting faculty about being an invert is inverting a situation, the motives and the roles.

Let's fast forward through a high-speed roadmap of discovery, from the endless and somewhat fruitless search for a father figure, to understanding the impact of being sexually abused as a child, to wanting to straighten the barbed wire around my motives to engage in consensual, negotiated, gradual, and controlled switching sexual and emotional interactions with other men: acts of amazing humiliation turning into worship, the Stockholm syndrome upside down, the transmogrification of pain, and the sadomasochistic Catholic dialectic, engorged and pulsating. Curse and gratitude exhaled under each breath as the bruised and welted flesh atones for the intolerance, hatred, disdain, and dread of contagion of others.

About that father figure search bit: it is a thirst that is never quenched. It creeps up and dries my mouth when a man thrusts; it signifies protection and care through penetration. Odd how some things that seem so dramatic in our thirties are accepted as part and parcel of life in the fifties. Now, it turns out the father I never had, and I always searched, lives within me: I have become the "queer daddy".

By 1994, I had almost forgotten Fernando and his milky adolescent ways. AIDS had materialized in every membrane, every sense, and every utterance from medics, in signed papers, charts, and each auscultation. Wretched aches, tensing, retching, my skin punctured a hundred times searching for collapsed veins, the war of radiation and chemo forging battles in every bend of my being. Clinics dispensed their drugs generously to stave off my writhing, vomiting, shitting, and crying. My pharmacological addiction began.

In London, Amsterdam, Seattle, New York, Toronto, San Francisco the cursed to die gargoyles gathered in dreadful covenants. I needed the dark, I needed the pain. I recall as if it were yesterday, descending on unsteady foot the steps down the catacomb of the Argos leather bar in the Amsterdam's *Warmoesstraat*. Down below, there was a cacophony of squeals, lashes, orders, pushing and shoving. Ritualized humiliation, performed slavery, rehearsed medicalization, piercing, spitting, choking, executed limit acts, the loss of dignity, all temporary and oddly freeing exorcisms that end in a sweet embrace, in a raspy throat uttering terms of endearment, a daddy, a boy, a friend, and a complete stranger entangled. That unintelligible hurt reversed every medical inspection, soothed the burning of my radiated skin, and overcame the fainting feeling, the nausea, the shortness of breath, the expiry date scribbled in my calendar.

This BDSM victory over clinical pain rarely makes the official records, or is even verbalized in the insincere institutional dialogue with clinicians. How do you explain a feeling and practice that defies health? Is it a niche market? Esoteric charlatanry? Acquired taste like sushi? Is BDSM a kind of purification of pain, a filtering of senses? Not everybody understands the dialectic of pain and humiliation and how sufferance cleanses, well...martyrs do, athletes do, ballerinas do, drug users do, and nuns do when flogging their pristine shoulders and breasts until they bleed. I still feel odd about talking about complementary and alternative medicine with my health care providers—never mind talking about sadomasochism!

Being an invert, the inversion and perversion, deviance, and obscenity come at a personal cost. Inversion and perversion awake the lying felines of fear and envy in many. Envy, jealousy, resentment, or jaundiced eye often comes in the capsule of an utterance, "I am clean and sober, you be too", in a widening of the pupils, or a squint of the eyes, and in the vortex of a condescending silence or indifference. We will not take you too seriously, we will call it TMI (too much information), we will expect until your own nervous giggle disavows you. *Pain is easy to identify. Envy is elusive.* Some have envied me that I came back to a full life, to a relationship, or a full career, after having crawled like an orphan at the doorstep of death and consumption – funny thing to envy. Others envied the public display, pleasure lives to be seen, to be performed. Envy lurches, swings out suddenly and stings. The moralist envies the whore, the mediocre hate self-possession.

And there is some poz envy, envy of the barebackers lurking there behind the self-satisfied liberated smirk. Envy comes in riding bareback the pink elephant in the room. There is music in the air in the night, the stars are bright, shining for you and me, Fernando.

I'm seen by a general practitioner every six months. From time to time, I see a specialist for my legs that sustained radiation damage forever, this lands me in a ER about 6 times a year with celulitis that has to be treated with IV antibiotics, I see a psychotherapist in an HIV mental health clinic to not drown in despair, I adhere to my SSRIs, I see a handsome specialist in anal dysplasia to prevent anal cancer. *Who would envy any of this seemingly fucked-up experience?* However, experience is a strange, nimble, intangible and coveted currency not wholesale in the globalized shopping malls. You can buy happiness, love, and health, and weapons, and war, but can't fake having lived it raw. For gay men, cock, that clownish little dangling appendage still leaks a powerful rivulet of intimacy, abnegation, and endurance in the name of love, or at least, in the name of abating loneliness for half an hour (or five minutes under a bridge).

This tale is not about HIV – the medicalization of a jungle of spirochaetes and bacillus and pathogens – *this tale is about sex with others, a way of living, and most importantly, a successful and powerful way of communicating with others* through body and fluids, through pregnant gestures, scenarios, clues, inversions of motives and action whimpers, whispers, rustles, lashes, stretching, slapping, soothing, clamps, fists, pistons, chokes, and risks – the industrial assembly line of extreme sex pioneered by western Caucasian men. I can't say the message of the medium is always affirmative, but it is loud. ABBA still rings in the inner ear, "now, we're old and grey Fernando". You may be a proud husband and father Fernando, or you became a soldier, a political refugee? Were you killed or disabled, or are you now forgetful and tremulous in Alzheimer's or Parkinson's? I will recall you always as the visiting archangel, the annunciation that something dark and amazing was marching deep into my life. Can you hear those drums Fernando?

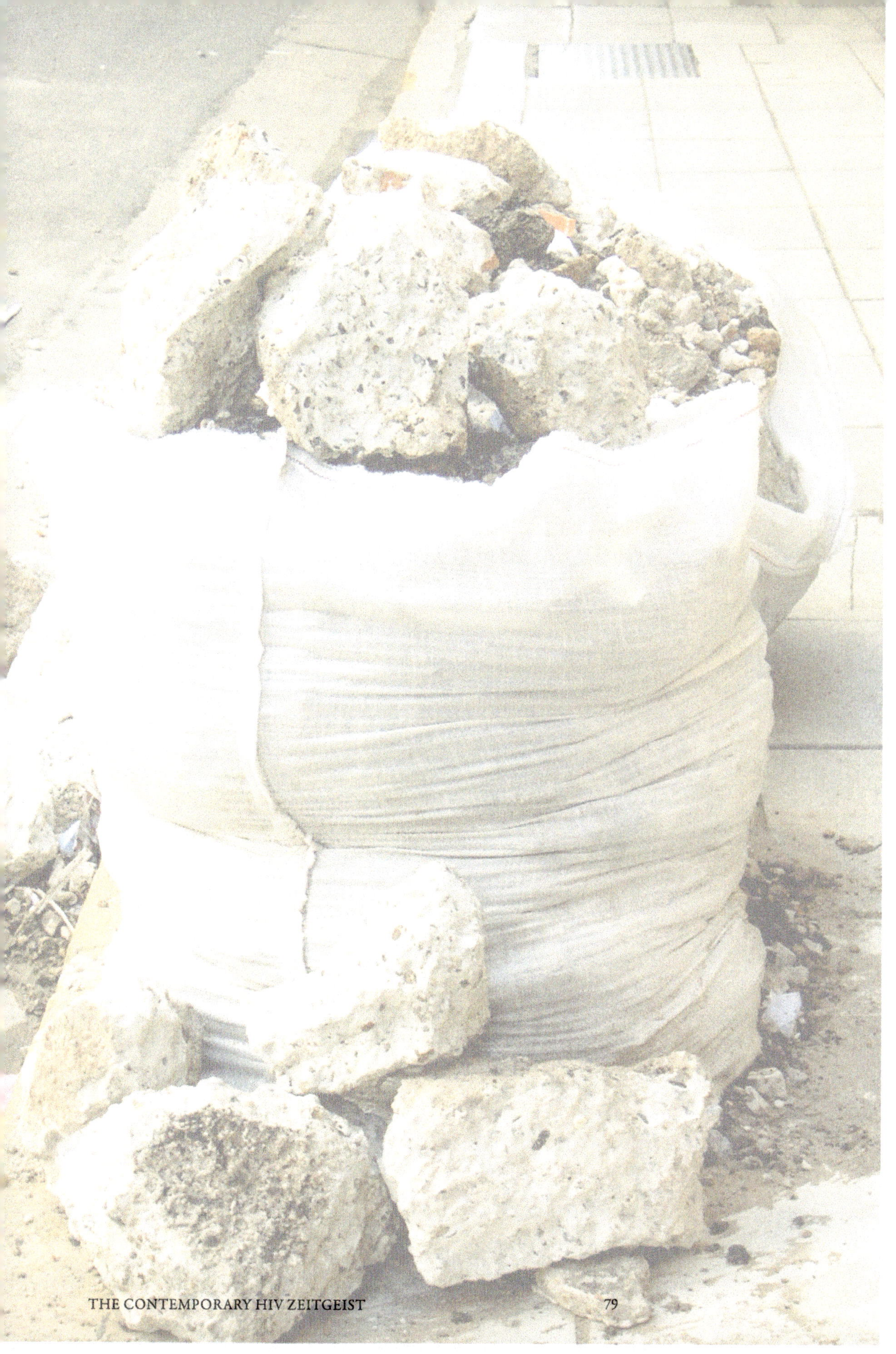

The Future Doctor's First Orgy

Gay group sex research envisioned through the lens of autoethnography.

Robert Birch

It's a warm, horny San Francisco night. I find a group sex party ad on Craigslist, and without hesitation I smoke some weed before ambling several blocks toward the Castro.

I've never been to an orgy before and the anticipation of the unknown makes my cock sweat inside my jeans. I find the house, a classic Bay area Victorian mansion. Two large gargoyles perch above black rod-iron gates leading into the old house. It's near Halloween.

I ring the doorbell half expecting Lurch from the *Munsters* to open a rust-hinged door and deep-croak, "You rang?" I step over the threshold and am welcomed instead by a nice older white cis guy standing behind a makeshift clothes check. He hands me a towel and a trash bag. I peel off the suggested donation, a greenback $20, wrapped around my Canadian driver's licence and credit card and start to undress. I jam the plastic cards and remaining bills into the toe of my suede cowboy boots, packing them in with the socks. I steal a look to see if the buffed-up grandpa thinks I'm paranoid. Beside me a small group of men mill about mostly nude. I'm tempted to ask them if they think my ass looks flat. I grin realizing its time to get over myself and suit down. I strip in the hall, shove my clothes in the green plastic garbage bag marked 107, suck in my gut and tuck in a towel that barely covers my 34 inch waist. I thank Mr. Coat Check and wonder how much I should tip him later. I avoid his seasoned gaze while playing the part of awkward newbie.

Barefoot, I feel the squish of decade-stained carpets and try not to think of foot rot. Not sure where to go I stand in an alcove and watch a few average looking guys pass through the curtain into what is obviously the darkroom. On the wall across from me is an old laminated map. It's called something like: A Geography of Sexual Desire. I'm relieved to focus on something and also encouraged to see how refreshing this community-made, grassroots sexual road map from the mid-80s is more relevant than any public health marketing campaigns I've seen in the last fifteen years. Drawn in a uniquely colourful hippy-esque aesthetic, the map is broken down into different terrains. The 'islands' are named for their repressions: *Internalized Phobias, Isolation,* and *Criticism of Other People's Kink.* The 'mainland' is defined by different states representing specific sexual acts: *Rimmington*, *Fuckfest*, *Fistlandia* etc. Behind the mountain range, non-consensual behaviours are hidden, implying that without mutual consent you damage someone else's sovereignty. I notice I am feeling safer in a way one- on-one safer sex discussions never feel. More relaxed, but not yet ready to brave the darkroom behind me I walk up a flight of stairs to the middle floor and step into a semi-nude kitchen potluck party already underway.

Big-bellied men balance paper plates on their guts while casually laying back on the couches. I'm told later that the second floor doubles as a meeting space for Monday night yoga. It's a different crowd tonight. These guys look like content regulars, chowing down and chatting after a busy day at the office or floral shop. I'm not as much turned off as thrown off by the food, soda pop, and the overall geniality of floor number two. Feeling a bit like an outsider I decide to move on.

A House of Healing Repute

As I walk up to the attic space I hear gently urging, honeyed electronic trance music. Turning the corner I take in the visual: a room full of erotic art including an extensive collection of cocks and other primitive erotic symbols. I realize the whole house is an homage to the phallus, with a liberal helping of what a regular later describes as "buttholes and beasty creatures". Baroque style stained glass windows illuminated with candles and other tastefully designed mood lighting makes for a quasi-sacred, snug space. The DJ is young; eyes to his vinyl, he sways to his own sermon.

In the middle of the room an art deco coffee table is covered inch for inch in pot and paraphernalia. The immediate contact high briefly transforms this instant other-worldliness into an oddly familiar domestic bliss. Sitting against the walls are men of varying ages with towels cascading over various body parts. Each man seems ready for some erotic touch yet distant to the opportunity beside him. Standing next to me, I turn to a dark, curly haired late-twenties guy wearing nothing but a hand-cut leather 'tool-belt' replete with condoms and lube. I compliment him on his very sexy self-care kit. "I made it myself," he says confidently. I introduce myself and ask him what's happening here. "This," he gestures in a way no else one notices, "This is the sexual rehabilitation zone." He's quiet and sincere, almost pragmatic. I look around again, momentarily seeing beyond my nerves to the scene before me. These men, mostly in their forties and fifties, black, white, Hispanic, Chinese. Part of their stoic beauty is entrenched in some deep isolation, aloneness still willing to risk connection, silently getting stoned with strangers, sharing sweet sounds and nursing desires as they fondle themselves, maybe each other. I thank Mr. Handsome and, while I am attracted to him I am unsure, somewhat unnerved, by this interim erotic space. He looks more sure of himself than I feel. I descend to the dungeon.

The Culture of Group Sex

Before I get my dick wet I want to introduce you, dear reader, to 'Darien', my 69 year-old fellow erotic adventurer. We've known each other for the past five years having met at an annual weeklong sex and intimacy retreat for gay men. Having lived in SF for decades he's a tough survivor living with a profoundly tenderized heart. He's also a regular at these parties. Darien delights in describing the 'tricked out' basement that includes a leather sling, fuck benches, beds, corners with carved out glory holes, and other dark spaces.

He's proud of this queer men's culture that offers a sliding scale from $12-20 with a NOTAFLOF policy ('no one turned away for lack of funds'). The house doubles as the host's private residence that he shares communally with roommates. "It's not commercial, more of a community kind of thing."

I ask about the history of the house. Apparently, the house was purchased to run weekly orgies as a radical service to the community. "It's slowed down significantly. Up until five years ago, (there was) a party weekly if not more. Lately, only Thanksgiving and Halloween, Pride, New Years party, every six to 12 weeks. The owner used to have another house in Oakland, 50 guys over for a weekend, big sexy orgy, a celebratory party. Swimming pools. Here, downtown, the numbers vary. Wall to wall, it used to be 200 men. You can tell from the bag count, it's shrunk to 50 guys."

A little whelmed by an image of all that cum, I ask Darien about sexual health at the parties. "It's a kind of environment where people negotiate safe sex, condoms everywhere. (It's an) understood sensibility that guys are either positive or they just don't care. If you approach somebody, then its like...it's sort of understood." I've run the gauntlet of my own disclosure strategies but as I'm about to tell him how I was unprepared for my own darkroom episode he interrupts and begins to explains the scene.

To Darien, and possibly many others, orgies are all about sharing communal erotic space: "There's a private/public dynamic. The first time I took my partner...we used to go to the baths, it took him a little while to get comfortable with the social and sexual. The first time can be uncomfortable....You learn how to read body language, comport yourself at that level. A bathhouse isn't personal... you pursue or grab, you respond to how they respond, groping in the dark. (At the sex party) there is a different sense of engagement. You want sex and, it's a bit of getting to that space of being more casual, not just treating others as sex objects but still having your desire fully present."

Get to Know the Scene Before Starring In It

My eyes adjust to the red lights. I see three ambitious bottoms scramble into position. Having sized me up they saddle up. Thigh by thigh, they mount their hungry haunches on a black leather bench. The guy closest to me gives his clean-shaven ass a shake to make sure he's got my attention. He does. They're lean cut late-thirties, good-looking cattle ready for market.

I approach the first little piggy and whisper in his ear, "Hi, you need to know I live with HIV." "Yeah, me too." I spit, slide my dick in him and begin to slowly rub his shoulders thinking I'm building up some rapport. "Fucking seed me, seed me." Whoa. Too fast, way too aggressive. I pull out.

I use his towel to clean off and move on to the next man. Repeat. "I'm Poz." He just whines and passively wiggles. Unsure of what else to do, I slap his ass and move on down the line. The third guy, having already overheard me pipes up, "We're all Poz here, now just fuck me."

I'm stopped. His rump's raw desire simultaneously makes my pre-cum dripping dick go limp and my goody-goody gay citizen hackles swell. There's no personal connection in these siloed fantasies. Obviously, it's dark. Nor can they see my bewilderment from their backsides. Nor do they want or need to. All of us naked with, but blinded to, one another's desire. I am just two minute dick for two minute ass. I exchange my barely used towel for the trash bag of clothes, dress and walk home.

Walk of Tame

I wish I had another joint. I ask myself whether I'm jealous of their self-abandon or just too over-stimulated to surrender to it. I want to believe they want what I do, to connect cock, ass and heart. I'm a not a fool because I'm hungry for both intensity and intimacy, just naïve to think I might experience it at my first orgy. I think to myself, "No one did anything wrong. We're all in a version of trying to figure it out alone, together...." I'm lying. My gut knows I'm still afraid of this dark I've been chasing for twenty-five years. Despite a cavalier approach to years of anonymous sex I'm still too pent up in my self definition/ defensiveness to surrender to tonight's Dionysian ecstatic ritual. I still desperately cling to my perpetual gay sunshine smile. In this self-dissolving space no socio-habitual trick has any currency. My good gay HIV disclosing boy receives no mercy here. Fucking in this dark means sacrificing my faggot shame in the alter of someone else's ass.

I pick up my pace in the now cooling late evening air. Similar to post-assault heroics, I flash on what I should have done. In my inner dungeon I see myself thrusting and growling, "Look me in the eye and let me fuck you like a real Poz fag!"

Stop. Slow down. Cigarette.

Watching the smoke dissipate I get that this sex space is about breaking down barriers, trespassing taboos; that's what I'm in for, starving to experience my own sexual r/evolution. My head knows I need role-relief from all the inherited social norms, the ceaseless hetero-pomp. In my heart I am not looking for romance so much as realness in my body. I really want to *share* a good fuck.

Another surge of violence. "Perhaps I should have dominated them, pushed their face down, make them meet *my* ultimatums." It passes.

Then the apology sets in. "I needed more –or better– or a combination of drugs..." This isn't self-pity; it's curiosity. No. It's pity trying to find its way to self-empathy. I turn the corner to see a jazz club spill out into the streets with people smoking, laughing, drinking. I stop to listen to what's happening outside of me.

Its impossible to feel down while walking the streets of this city. I turn, reposition my blue balls and bruised veracity. I put out the cigarette, hike up my jacket collar; I walk, lean deeper into my desires, sensing how they both shape and hollow me. I know sex wounds. It has also, if only in rare, vulnerable times, healed. Talking to myself right now helps. For the moment I can rest. I've proven that I am willing to take risks to explore an erotic edge. No one asks for proof of risk (unless you are a Poz person defending yourself in a court of law). Give it a rest, ~birch. No, not my style.

A friend suggests I often seek the erotic salve while willing to risk the injury. Ecstasy is the only remedy that makes any sense to me. The ecstatic liberates the living from the dead. The call to orgies is a call to immanence.

When I follow my desire, trust the animal of myself, I'm going to confront the animal in you. The non-verbal butt sniffing is hot. The ritual of it feels necessary, revitalizing. Eye contact lets you know how I'm seeing you. It takes confidence to work up a lather of lust together. I want to know how you play with vulnerability – mine and yours – and how you show up in the foreplay. But those were my one-on-one rites.

What's new to me now is the party itself. Checking out how people work each scene, each floor, requires its own unique social skill set. Small talk in the kitchen, a toke and a massage on the top floor, bring a friend next time, whatever it takes to get me out of my own head trip. If I want orgiastic randomness and ecstatic abandon I need to pay attention to what I bring to the party. To begin, I need to remember that it's a party.

This particular sex party is clearly more than a cum dump. While I cut short my initial experience I reflect on what my weathered elder, Darien, says about sexual community. I couldn't register what was going on because I'd never experienced, let alone imagined, a truly communal scene. If *how* I see the world mostly determines *what* I see, then obviously my frame of reference shapes my outcomes. I'm willing to risk a new erotic world view for a more fulfilling and potentially healing sex adventure.

That leather tool kit man really turned me on. His DIY safer sex style was miles ahead of my verbal consent failures. What stopped me from engaging more with this beautiful, creative man? In part I couldn't get past my old condom narrative. I saw function where he was showing up with a new form of playing. If I'm going to play in a new way I need to finish off my late 80s sex panic, not just outride it. Also, I brought my compensatory anonymous sex bathhouse story with me to the party. Communal sex is obviously more than a looping porno tape in the head. Perhaps if I spent more time chatting over food or chilling out with the cute DJ, I would have relaxed into the offering, not just the taking. The opening might have shown up with handmade tool belt guy. I bet he was a gracious, full throttle lover. Not deterred, I'll get my orgy on at some point. While the notion of an erotic healing quest may be more than many will stomach, there's a new kink to be discovered hanging out in the attic of sexual rehabilitation. Time together is needed to re-imagine what kind of lover one wants and wants to be. In these shared erotic spaces there's a liminal flesh sharing world that exists beyond viral designations. When I'm ready. Group sex has secrets of surrender to share.

Post-prescription

Weeks after my first group sex event I got a call from a close friend leaving his job at a regional Canadian AIDS service organization. He asked me to apply for the position of the gay men's outreach worker. I refused. He then asked me to facilitate a weekend community event for gay cis/trans men. I agreed. It's a great feeling of coming home to community.

I quickly learned how stagnant the mainstream state of gay men's health has been since the indescribable relief provided by HAART (Highly Active Antiretroviral Therapy, the meds). I've also long noticed that gay men don't talk about healing nor emotional health anymore.

After a short two-year stint in an ASO (AIDS services organization), I was invited to pursue a PhD. I said to my husband, "Shoot me if I say yes." Now in my second year of a doctoral program I'm researching group sex events, what epidemiologists call high-risk, MSM (man on man) sex and substance use environments. My friend and co-editor, Marcus Greatheart, instantly dubbed me Dr. Orgy. Through the laughter I tapped into the idea of launching Dr. Orgy's Pleasure Emporium on positivelite.org, an award winning online HIV/AIDS magazine. Some people kindly confided in me that I wouldn't be taken seriously, be seen as legitimate in the field of gay men's health as a result. I got scared and stuck. I shut up and therefore shut down. For the past six months I stopped writing – not a smart move for a graduate student. This article is therefore, with all due respect, another iteration of coming out. I am a researcher, a 'participant' and uncompromisingly, someone who knows how the arms of a community of lovers actually feels.

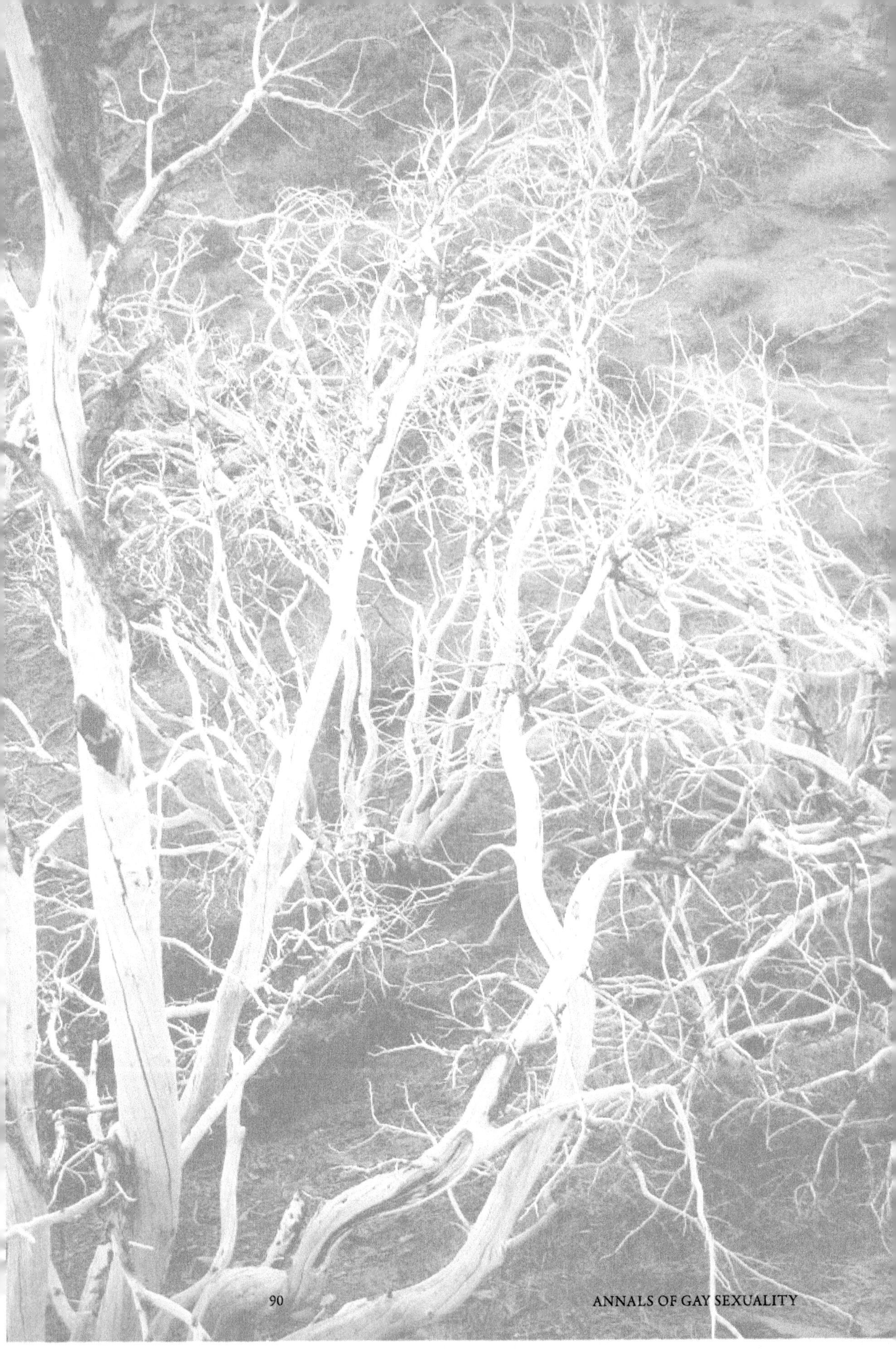

OVER PAGE:

BELIEVE IT OR NOT, THERE WAS A TIME IN MY LIFE WHEN I DIDN'T GO AROUND ANNOUNCING I WAS A FAGGOT. | WES FANELLI

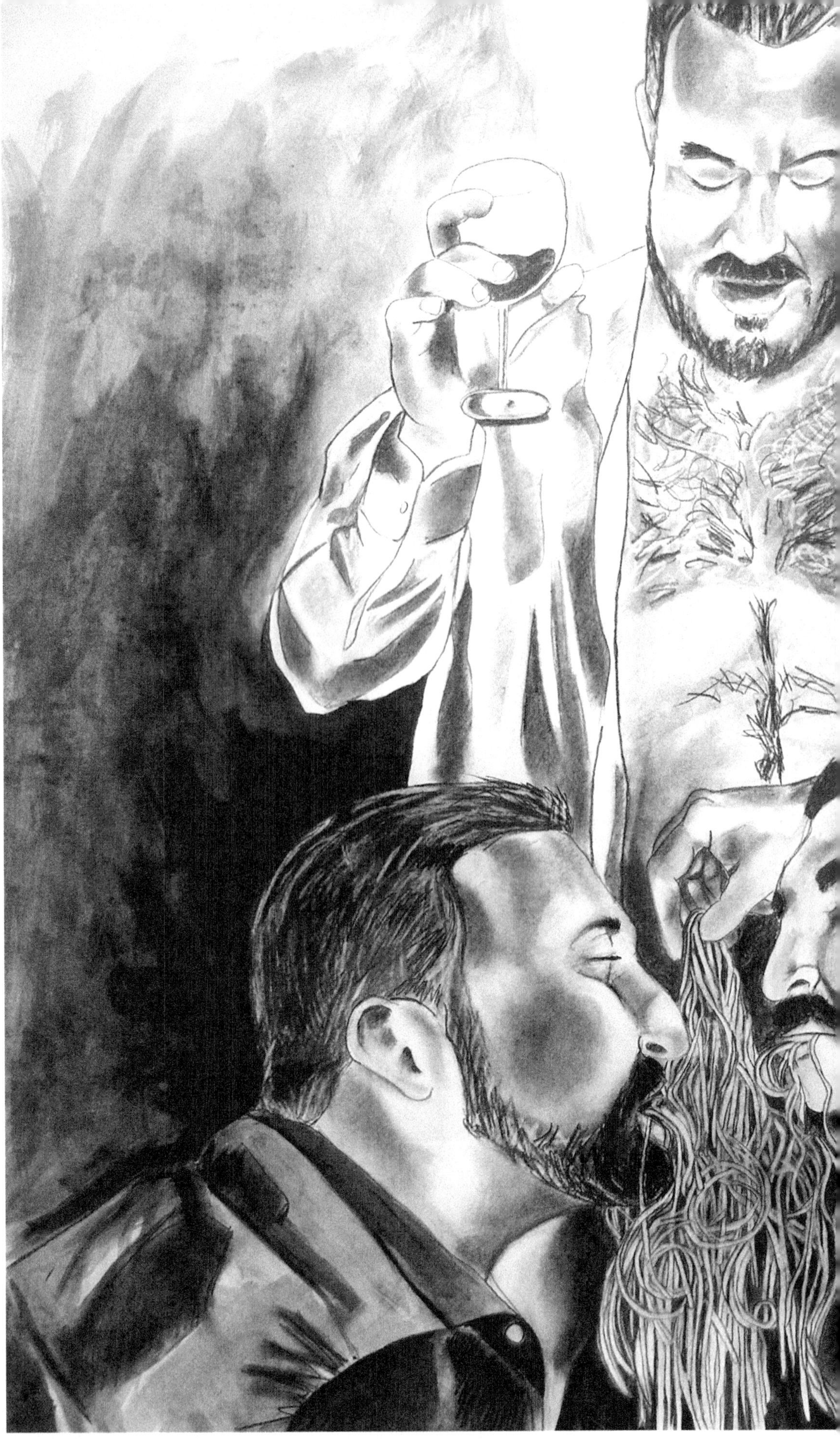

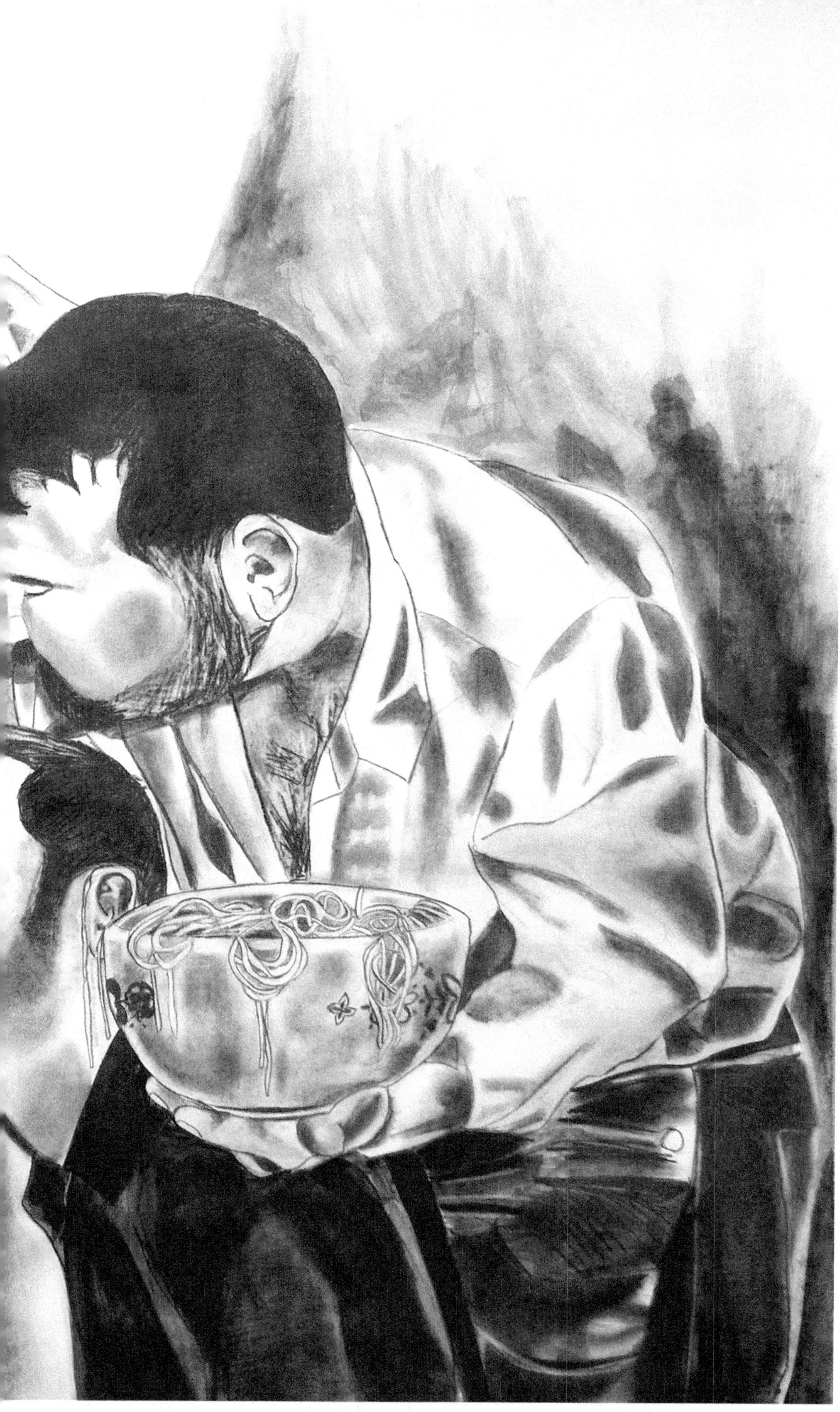

See Dick Fuck.

Mischief with
Marcus Greatheart

Gordon—
with love and
gratitude for
the chat that started
this whole project!
[illegible]

Marcus:

Mischief is beside me in bed. He's one of my dearest friends and we sleep well together. Like many of my good gay friends (and their friends, and their friends), we dated and were intimate before shifting to friendship.

It's just after Christmas 2013 and we're guests of my co-editor Birch and his handsome husband Mark. I'm on two weeks' vacation from school and my brain wants to think about anything but Medicine.

An hour earlier, as we snuggled under the wool blankets, I confessed to him my jealousy of the sexual liberation he has as an undetectable (HIV-positive) gay man, from my own place of sero-negativity. This was in response to a tale he'd shared of a fuck buddy coming over for a 30-minute shag where spit replaced lube, and condoms were unnecessary between two ser-positive men. The simplicity and - let's face it - erotic strength of the narrative left me hot and bothered on multiple levels.

That's the night we agreed to start a conversation about what it means to live our (sex) lives.

Mischief:

I don't really like condoms. I never have. For most of my life, for one reason or another, I've never needed to use condoms. When I started having multiple partners, condoms were pretty awkward and many times I didn't use them.

Now that I'm undetectable, I no longer worry about contracting the virus. Given the recent research, I'm also less worried about passing on the virus. I'm a chronic discloser of my HIV status, and I prefer condomless sex. For me, sex without a condom is less complicated and frankly fuckin' hot.

Your jealousy of my sexual freedom is warranted.

Marcus:

HIV has been a constant in my life (in general) and sex life (in specific) since I came out in the mid-1980s. It's always there in the bedroom (and other locales) because it comes with so many accoutrements: condoms and lube for certain and other toys depending on the scene.

Guilt is probably my worst enemy with regard to HIV. I've survived this long as a neg guy that it somehow seems foolish to consider HIV-positivity.

I sense a chasm between us.

Mischief:

I agree. When I was negative, like you, I was always super concerned about HIV. Today, I rarely think of it. In fact caring for my teeth takes more time and effort than caring for my HIV.

Marcus:

As a healthcare provider and future physician, I wanted to explore the reasons for staying HIV-negative through this dialogue with Mischief. There are bureaucratic and logistical reasons for remaining HIV-negative at the moment. But hypothetically, if a gay male patient sat across from me were to ask why he should worry about sero-converting, what would my argument be?

Research published recently states that an urban, white, gay male who acquires the HIV virus today in a resource-rich jurisdictions and begins HAART is expected to have basically the same life expectancy as someone who remains negative. There are some potential side effects to the medications but, anecdotally, many of my friends on these meds experience none. I appreciate this line of inquiry comes with much privilege attached, and does not reflect the reality for many marginalized groups, but hear me out.

At what point will HIV medications become equivalent to blood pressure meds: another treatment of lifestyle choices? Except, rather than high salt diets and red meat as contributing factors, the choice was sex without a condom. Some research suggests HIV-positive people might even be healthier due to access to regular healthcare, monitoring of blood work, and free or low-cost complementary therapies in many major centres.

Some might also argue that the reduced anxiety that comes with no longer being worried about contracting HIV (you already have it) makes life easier. The dating pool of healthy, happy and well-adjusted poz men is presently well stocked. And, if a guy limits sex to those who are similarly positive then the legal ramifications of disclosure are arguably moot.

Mischief:

Before the advent of PrEP, an HIV-negative friend who was having lots of condomless sex asked me that very question you fear: why should he worry about sero-converting. I answered honestly, and given what you and I have both said, I didn't do a great job of convincing him to stay negative. A year after he sero-converted I asked him if he regrets his decision. He didn't.

The reasons to stay negative weren't that compelling to him. The cost of HIV care was a moot point; here in British Columbia the cost of treatment is not borne by the individual. The (minor) inconvenience of meds was moot; today he'd likely be on PrEP. The potential side effects and long-term health implications of treated HIV; also moot.

My most compelling argument was, and remains: the stigma attached to being HIV-positive.

Marcus:

The discourse around 'HIV envy' speaks to ongoing and significant stigma that, frankly, many of my poz friends no longer endorse. Lack of side effects from once-a-day medications and improved healthcare means they are working, contributing members of society; nowadays fewer poz guys are living on social assistance or disability. And the divide between poz and neg guys is, it appears, an artifact of the past as younger gay and queer men are much less invested in AIDS history.

The division becomes hazy.

The arguments are no longer as strong and, unless a flaw in treatment emerges, or the 'super virus' of urban mythology finally appears, then we may remain the haves and have nots.

And with the heightened focus on HIV, many of us were less concerned about the other sexually transmitted infections. And I don't think that health educators, myself included, did an effective job of conveying how infection with an STI increased vulnerability to HIV. As an HIV educator since the early 1990s, I've often said that God (insert name of any Higher Power here) never intended for a condom to be a part of anyone's sex. A barrier prevents the flow of fluids, causes friction and leaves a bad taste. There may be wisdom for some to use condoms in certain situations, but that doesn't mean they're intended to be there.

Mischief:

The effect HIV has had on my life has been rather minimal. Granted there was a dismal three-year period when I first sero-converted. I was not on meds, I watched my health decline quite rapidly, I was super infectious, and I didn't feel great about myself. I'm a huge proponent of the new approach to starting meds immediately.

Today, I'm on triple therapy. My viral load is undetectable (<40 copies of the virus per milliliter of blood). Recent research is showing that it's next to impossible for me to pass on the virus (passing on the virus was a huge fear for me and most HIV+ guys). I'm not immuno-compromised (my CD4 count recently surpassed 1,200 and the range for a healthy person is 410-1,330). I have a fantastic physician (and just finding a physician is difficult for an HIV-negative guy nowadays). I have free access to complementary therapies like massage, counseling, support groups, acupuncture, nutrition counseling, and the like.

Marcus:

A new tide has turned.

Pre-Exposure Prophylaxis (PrEP), a seemingly effective antiviral geared toward HIV-negative people, is now available in many jurisdictions. Just this week the CDC recommended its use among gay men and other higher risk populations. The typical arguments against were thrown out to the media, most specifically that use of PrEP will necessarily lead to increased STI rates and possibly perpetuate antibiotic-resistant strains. The underlying assumption is that condom use will stop completely, but current evidence does not support that assertion.

To be clear, I don't believe that every gay man should be on PrEP. Instead, I believe it's indicated for those at highest risk: guys in relationships with poz guys, and those who are inconsistent with condom use with partners whose sero-status they can't be assured is negative. Some might even argue that unprotected sex with an undetectable man is safer and while I support that theoretically, I can't say that I would do it.

Marcus:

The benefit of PrEP is not solely in the reduction HIV infection risk, which is stated to be approximately 99 percent effective in those who are adherent to daily use. It also requires the individual to attend their Family Doctor's office every three months for repeat HIV testing and STI screening. I would argue that this increased surveillance and concordant treatment will also impact STI levels in that new infections are treated more quickly then had these individuals been tested and treated symptomatically or as part of regular annual preventative health screening. Add to this the regular surveillance of known HIV-positive men on HAART which should include STI screening and conceivably we could make a significant reduction in STI incidence.

Mischief:

If I were still negative today, I'd be annoyed that the health department isn't paying for PrEP.

Marcus:

The jury is still out.

Undetectable. Positive. Living with AIDS. Multiple identities defined by particular lab blood work, but so disparate in experience on many levels.

Mischief tells me he's undetectable. He's not HIV-positive or living with AIDS. He's part of a newer breed who sero-converted in recent years and started treatment quickly. He tells me his dating life improved after he started disclosing more publicly his status on online profiles. Guys he'd been into for a while admitted they were also poz and felt it was too much bother and worry to date a neg guy, so they didn't. He was like a southern girl at a coming out cotillion and, man, was his dance card full.

MISCHIEF:

You talk about my full dance card when I first sero-converted, the well stocked pool of undetectable guys and negative guys being more open to condomless sex with undetectable guys. While there is an element of truth to all of these, one cannot discount the effect of stigma.

It's pretty easy to find a quick bareback fuck. There are guys online that seek me out for being undetectable, and when I disclose to guys at the bathhouse, their reply is usually 'no condom, right?' When it comes to dating, however, I find it a bit more difficult.

I put the {+} in my Scruff profile because I am tired of rejection. Often, once I disclose, the conversation ends abruptly. I have much better reception from Gen-Y guys: some of them are clueless about HIV; others are very educated and unafraid of undetectable guys. But Gen-Y guys are at least a decade younger than me, and I'm far from a daddy.

I prefer to date in my cohort: the Gen-Xers. Many of the neg Gen-X and older guys sero-sort: that is, they only date other neg guys. I also prefer condomless sex, and would rather take HIV out of the equation by sero-sorting.

When it comes to dating other poz, or undetectable, Gen-X guys it's a pretty bleak scene. First, I refuse to date a guy who only has sex on chems (meth or other drugs) – that rules out a good portion of the men. From those left over, we need to eliminate the guys who are unavailable for dating – because they're already in relationship, or have given up in frustration (like I've done many times). It took about three years of repeated disappointment, but I've finally started dating a fantastic guy, and I'm doing my best to keep him around.

Marcus:

Poz-envy and sero-negativity.

This is a conversation set among a particular Zeitgeist in gay men's culture. As a group of us in our later 30s to 50s grow older at a time of particular advances in the medicine of HIV. Where treatment is prevention. Where in Canada and other jurisdictions, the medications are available from the health authority and paid by the government. We're obviously privileged in Canada with universal healthcare. And in British Columbia particularly, we benefit from the knowledge generated in the AIDS machine that is the BC Centre for Excellence in HIV/AIDS.

Mischief:

I might like to whine but I do know that I receive great care. I'm privileged.

Right: Clean /Dirty |
Grahame Perry

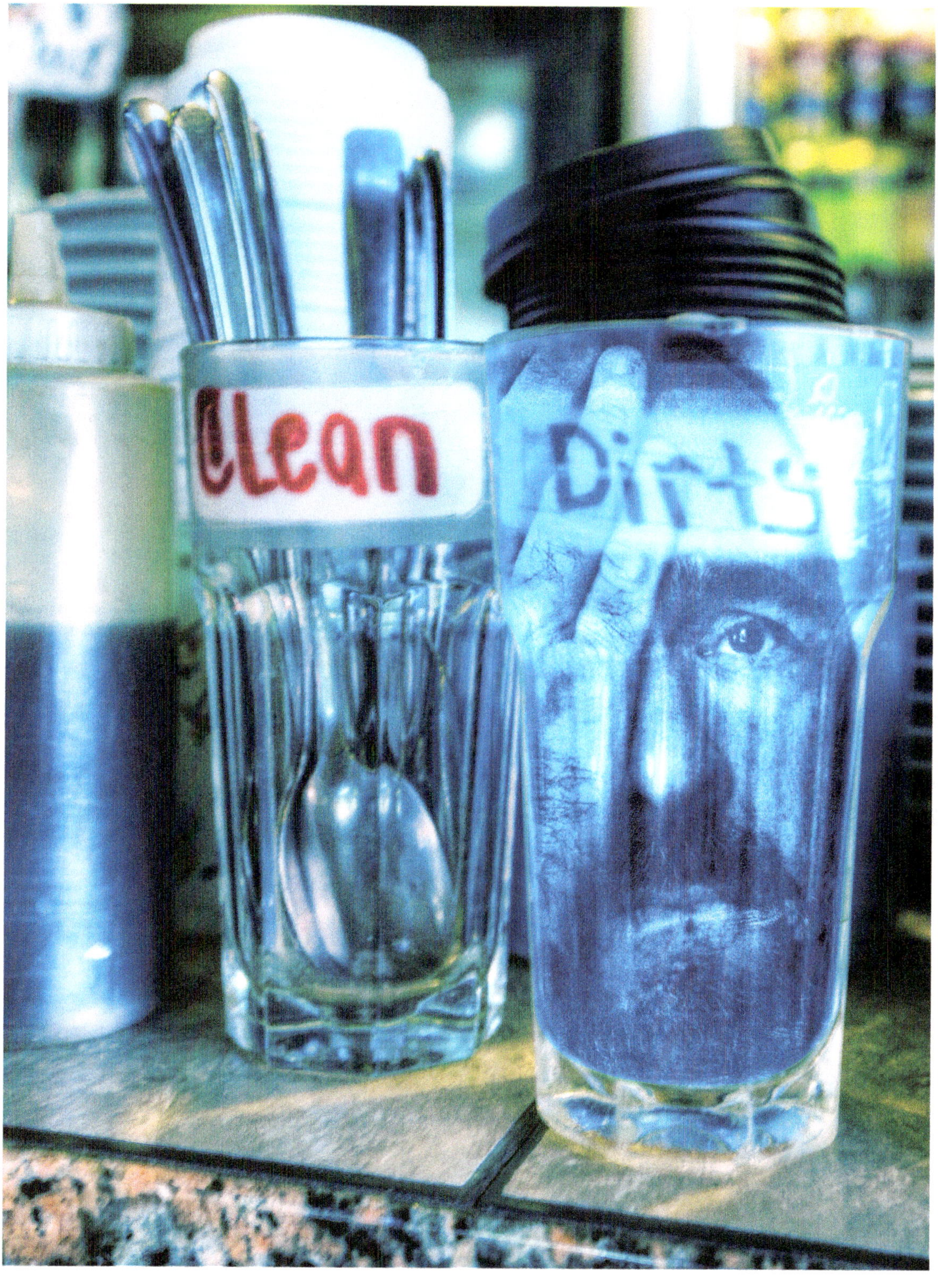
Clean
Dirty

How Can You Be Beautiful To Me?

Timothy D. Rains

I put my hand on your chest,
to see if your heart is still beating,
and I hear you,
your heart is still beating, I can feel,
it pulsing when I desire,
to put my hand on your chest,
how can you be so beautiful to me,
in body, and spirit, sculpted,
so beautiful to me, of body, and spirit,
and yet, when I put my hand to your chest,
your heart stops beating, and I hear you,
pulsing, but I can't feel,
your heart beating, how are you still beautiful,
to me, still beautiful, when I desire,
to put my hand on your chest,
in your body, in your spirit, sculpted desire,
in my hand, putting in your body,
in your spirit, desire, sculpted, beautiful to me,
and yet I can't feel your heart beating, and
I wonder if you were always this beautiful,
to me, always this beautiful, to him, to me,
to him, and did he put his hand upon your chest,
to hear your heart beating, to hear your heart pulsing,
did he desire to hear your heart beating,
to hear your heart desire, and is he the reason
your heart no longer beats in body, in spirit,
in body, because you were beautiful to him,
and him, and him, and him, and him, and him,
and in your body, in your spirit, in your desire,
you were beautiful, in your body, in your spirit,
in your desire, you were beautiful, but you couldn't
stop him, stop you, stop him, stop you,
from putting his hand upon your chest, in your body,

in your spirit, in your desire for him, and him, and him,
and you, to stop you and him, and him and you,
but you were beautiful, you were beautiful, you are,
beautiful, in body, in spirit, in desire, and
I desire, your spirit, your body, to put my hand,
on your chest, and feel your heart beating,
but I am afraid, I won't be able to stop,
the desire, to put my hand upon your chest,
and feel your heart pulsing, feel your heart beating,
feel my heart pulsing, feel my heart beating,
feel my desire, in body, in spirit, in body, in desire,
in heart, pulsing, beating, pulsing, desire, like you,
stop.

OVER PAGE:

Touch | Pan

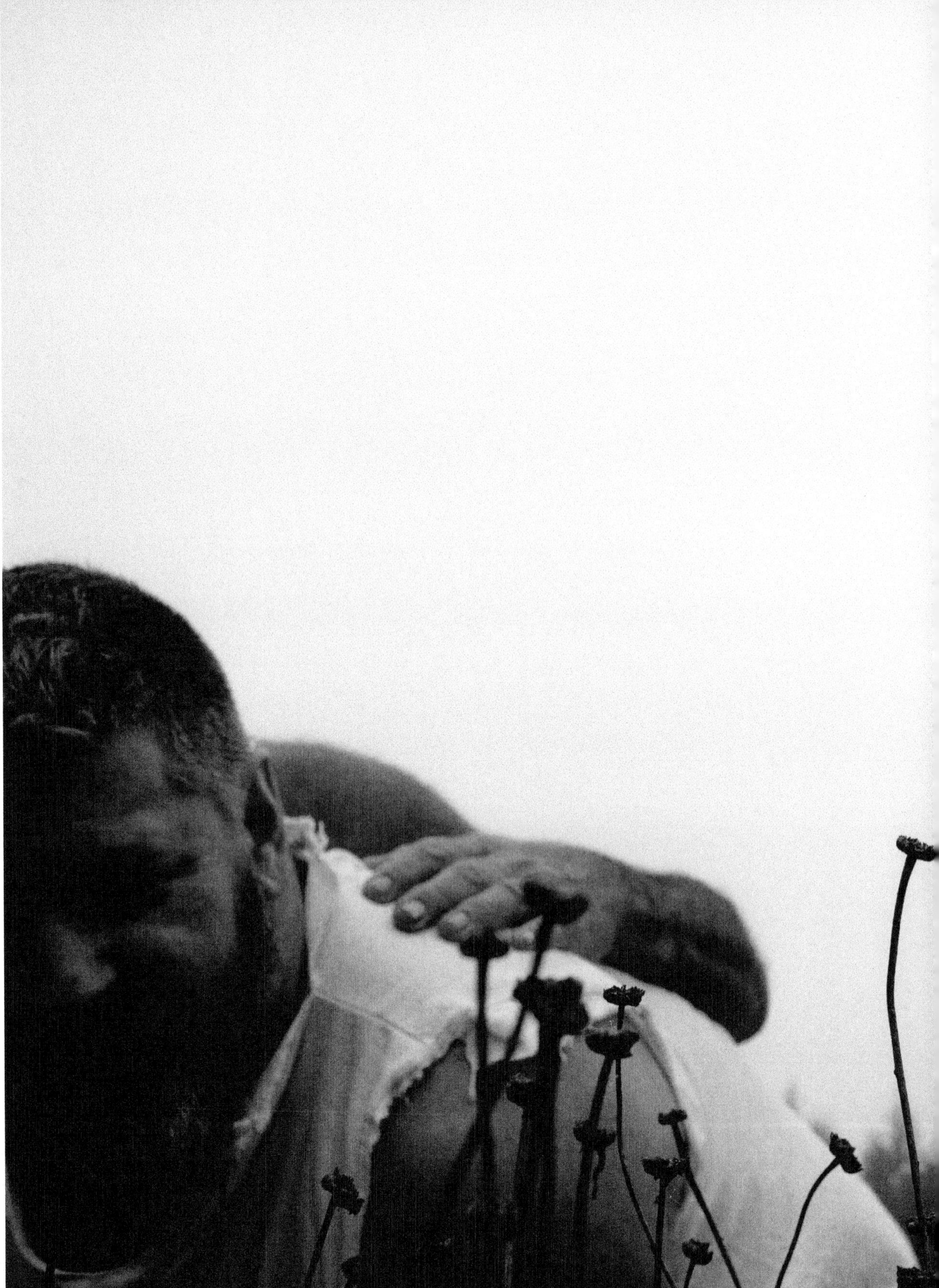

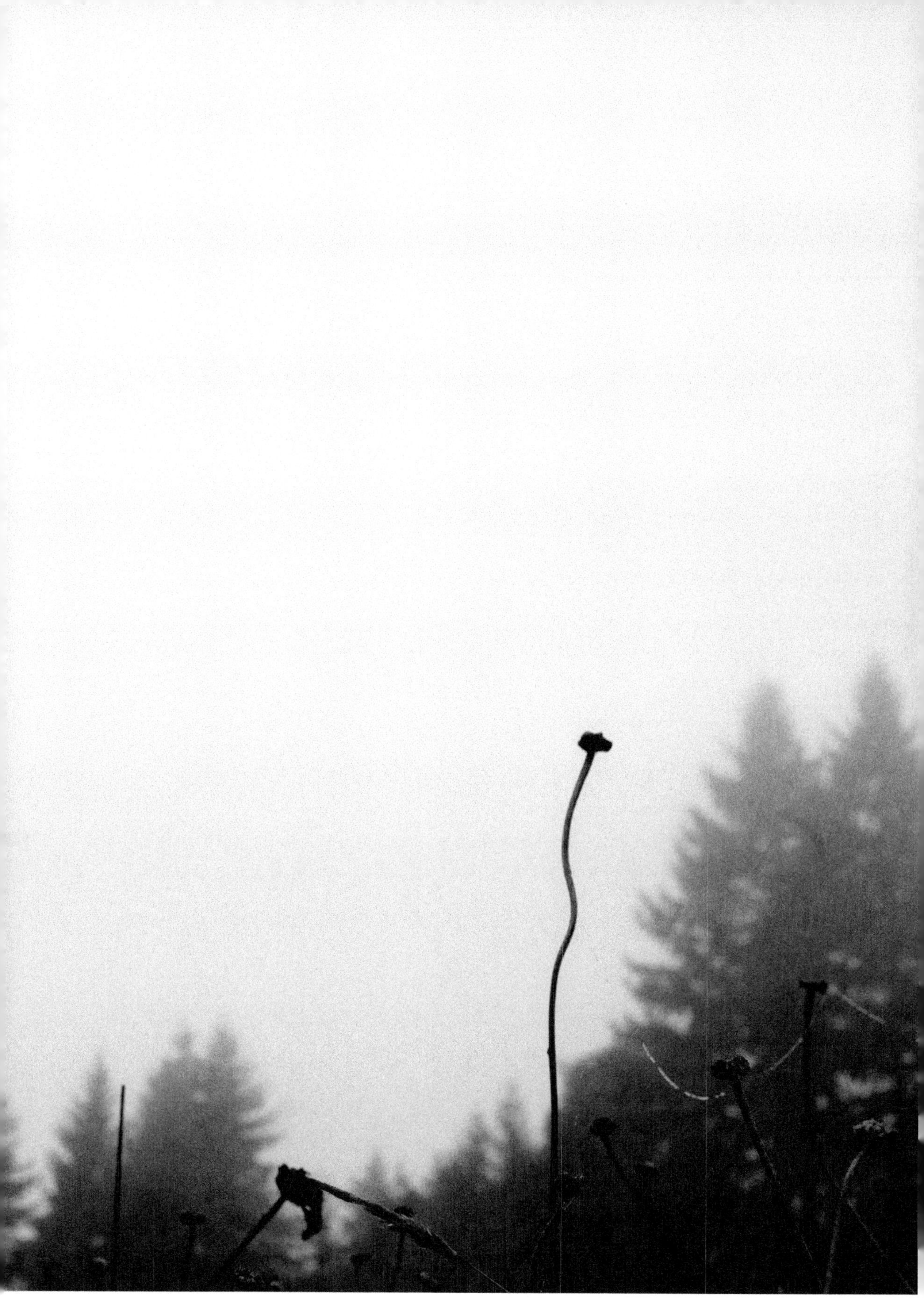

Barebacking

Simon Sheppard

In the beginning, you didn't mean to. Not at all. But there you were, with a condom around your rapidly deflating dick and a beautiful brown Indian man in your bed. The Indian's hole was, as usual, tight, and the guy had already told you that he'd thought you two had fucked raw before, a few months back. Which wasn't true. Whatever.

You were virtually certain your partner was negative; you knew damn well that you yourself were. You peeled off the condom and threw it on the floor. Squirting a little more lube on your dick, you began sliding your hard-on against the man's warm, welcoming ass. Your cock instantaneously grew hard, harder than it had been all night.

It had been so many years, so long since you'd had unprotected sex. The Indian guy turned over on his stomach, the way he always liked to get fucked.

It was easy, amazingly easy, to slip inside. For the first time since you'd started screwing the guy, it seemed like there was no resistance, no fight. This is so wrong, you thought, but that didn't stop you from sliding all the way in and staying there. Considering the number of times you had fucked the fellow—a married man whose wife (pronounced, in the Indian fashion, "vife," providing a little cross-cultural thrill) was often out of town—this time felt surprisingly unfamiliar. Luxurious, that was the word for it. *Luxurious.*

You raised yourself up on your extended arms and looked down at the broad brown back. Sliding your dick in and out, in and out, you couldn't believe how totally, absolutely, fantastically great it felt.

Well, strictly speaking, that wasn't true. You *could* believe it, easily. It was, after all, how sex had once been supposed to feel, but at the same time it was as if the two of you had a dirty little secret, one neither of you would ever tell.

The Indian man had always been, in fact, a great, hungry bottom once his hole had loosened up. But now, skin on skin, there had been no initial tightness, no gradual ramping up of pleasure, and it took an effort of will not to come too soon. You would have liked to switch positions, to get the guy on his back, look down at his handsome face, kiss him. But it was what it was: The guy didn't kiss, and he preferred it from behind. So you pounded away, enjoying what surely must be a once-only raw fuck.

You were so very, very happy.

"You're not going to come inside me, right?"

"Of course not." You didn't mention you'd already felt yourself leaking precum deep inside his hole.

Pretty soon you sensed you were reaching the point of no return. "I'm gonna come," you said, pulling your slick cock out of the well-used hole, looking down to watch the naked shaft sliding out. Without even having to touch yourself, you shot off all over the man's back, milky sperm on chocolate skin. You caught your breath, then rolled off your partner.

The just-fucked man turned over, a big smile on his face. His dark cock was still fully hard. He reached down and stroked himself till his nutsack, nearly black, tightened, pumping a big load out onto his belly.

"I loved when you fucked me," the man said, afterwards. He had never used the word "love" before, in any context.

"Me, too," you said. "A lot." *I won't be doing that again,* you thought.

*

On your way home from the Indian's, the warm spring night seemed full of possibilities, the fragrance of night-blooming jasmine, for once, not cloying but absolutely perfect.

You stopped into an all-night donut place, braving the fluorescents, and got an apple fritter, still hot out of the oven, and a cup of coffee. The caffeine would keep you up till dawn, but that was okay; no work the next day. You bit into the smooth, sweet dough. Life was, indeed, good.

If you *had* done something dangerous, you had no idea what it had been.

*

A couple of weeks later, after you'd fucked your buddy a couple of more times, both without a condom, the Indian man's wife returned and further fucking was, for the moment, off. Even your e-mails went unanswered.

For a week or so after that, unmanageably horny, you jacked off two or three times a day, but one night you decided to throw caution pretty much to the winds and answer an ad you'd seen online.

When your correspondent came over, he was even better looking than he'd looked in the photo he'd e-mailed—a very pleasant surprise. In his mid-twenties, the guy's face was pretty and unlined, his hair long and blondish, his handlebar mustache a waxed-up architectural achievement that framed his big, soft-looking lips.

"My name's Marc, with a 'c,'" he said.

You hadn't even gotten to the bedroom when you started tearing each other's clothes off. Marc, sensing a belt-unbuckling problem, undid his own jeans and pulled them halfway down, revealing blue-checked boxers.

It was gratifying, when you reached down and groped through the cotton fabric, to discover that Marc's cock was small, thin, and very hard. Contrary to what you supposed you were supposed to prefer, you in fact had a thing for little dicks, and it was exciting to you that this lovely, slightly overweight young man had one.

Once Marc had thoroughly stripped down, his body plump, a bit furry, and otherwise desirable, it turned out that he also had an edible-looking, perfectly pink hole.

"Get on the bed, on your back, legs up," you said, and once Marc had done exactly that, hands grabbing ankles to keep his legs in the air, you hungrily dived right in. You really loved eating ass. Loved it past the point of explanation, of reason. Even at the height of your caution, you'd always rimmed asses—and, amazingly, had never suffered more than an upset tummy as a result of your passions.

After you'd sated yourself, you backed off, wiped your mouth, and spit-lubed your dick. This time, unlike the first bare fuck with the Indian, there was no hesitation. Marc had advertised for a raw fuck, and a raw fuck was what he was going to get.

He had warned you by e-mail that his hole was tight, but it wasn't, not really, though in any case, the extended rimming had prepped it well. Just a little prodding, and there it was: the feeling of skin sliding against skin. Well, it was against mucous membrane really, but that sounded a lot less romantic, and with your dick all the way inside Marc, your pubic bone pressing up against the boy's meaty ass, you weren't about to quibble over terminology.

"I'm getting a cramp in my leg," Marc said.

"Want to ride me, instead?"

"Sure."

You rearranged yourselves, Marc on top and straddling you, hole against hard cockhead. With one swift stroke, Marc lowered himself down on you, velvety hot softness enveloping your sensitive shaft.

You looked up at Marc's handsome face, at the cute mustache, the bright blue eyes, the skinny little dick oozing precum, and though you knew you were expected to keep fucking for a good long time, you realized you were, distressingly, already at the point of no return.

"Fuck, I'm going to come," you said.

If Marc was disappointed, he hid it well. "Go for it," he encouraged.

"Inside?" It had been prearranged, so you didn't really need permission, or if you did, it was your own permission to yourself.

"Yeah."

The spasms came from deep inside his balls, and they lasted for a long, long time, until you'd shot your entire load of sperm inside Marc's furry ass. Marc leaned over, allowing your dick to slide out of his hole. Though he'd said in his e-mails that he didn't kiss, Marc planted a surprising soft kiss on your mouth; that moustache felt great.

"Can I ask you a favor, Marc?"

"Sure, I think."

You'd been wanting to do this for a decade, more. "Let me eat your ass a little more."

When Marc was obligingly on all fours, you kneeled behind him and spread his asscheeks. As the hole relaxed, a stream of cum trickled out. You plunged your tongue against it, licking it up.

You jerked away with a shudder. *What the fuck am I doing?* you thought. Then you relaxed, snuggled your face against Marc's ass, and slurped some more.

*

Like any loss of virginity, you reflected, the first time had been the hardest. (Though okay, it hadn't really been the first time, since you had, many years ago, never used rubbers at all.)

But now that you had become almost accustomed to barebacking, nearly reconciled, now that you had found the very perfect Marc, the blond boy wasn't answering your e-mails; you sent four intentionally breezy notes suggesting you meet up again, then, not wanting to seem a pest, not wanting to feel any more rejected than necessary, gave up.

You once had an English boyfriend who'd taught you the phrase, "In for a penny, in for a pound." Though the Euro had made it technically obsolete, in this case it seemed appropriate.

A barebacking party was not, in your city, hard to find.

*

You hadn't been to a sex party for years, not, in fact, since you'd brought home a persistent case of scabies. So it was with a certain amount of trepidation that you made your way to the address specified in his invitation.

You were still unsure, actually, just what you'd be prepared to do once you got to the party. Unlike the Indian man and unlike Marc, the men at the party, you assumed, were more likely to fuck first, negotiate afterwards. Still, it might be interesting just to walk into the party....

When you paid your entrance fee and walked in the door—of a nicely furnished, middle-class house, as it happened, not some sleazy dive—you were pleasantly surprised to find a goodly variety of men already there, some already naked. Out of the couple of dozen guys, there were a few standard-issue gym bunnies, an unclothed older man with a thatch of unexpectedly sexy gray hair on his meaty chest, a young Asian man, Thai maybe, with beautiful eyes and a tight-fitting lycra wrestling singlet that showed off his hard dick. A prodigiously tattooed, skinny young blond guy with piercings everywhere, including his dick, a black man in Bermuda shorts, a bear or two. And you.

There was an air of sociability mixed with awkward expectancy; some of the men seemed to know each other well, while others hung around on the margins. Then one guy, obviously the organizer/host, announced that the door had been closed to newcomers and detailed the rules for the evening.

You hadn't realized till then what the set-up actually was—insufficient research, you supposed. The party was in fact a gang-bang, the tattooed boy the planned recipient of everyone else's loads. This was not only not a turn-on for you—you'd planned on a one-on-one, or a three-way at most—but a little worrisome, too. Fucking one ass without a rubber was one thing, plunging your cock into a reservoir of other men's cum, much of it no doubt infected, quite another. It was only after the festivities were already underway that you realized you might have asked to go first, thereby shortening your participation but allaying your fears. By then, though, one of the gym bunnies had groaningly popped a load inside the tattooed boy's ass, his cock quickly replaced by the gray-haired man's.

Meanwhile, some of the men were getting blown—fluffed for their upcoming fucks, no doubt, since oral sex to completion was not the main dish on the menu. The muscular man who just finished fucking was headed your way, his cock still hard, at least probably a testament to the powers of Viagra.

“"Drop your pants and I'll blow you," the muscular man said.

With a shock, you realized that you were the only one there who was still fully clothed. You unzipped your fly, took out your half-erect cock, and, when the well-built man was on his knees, slipped it between the guy's lips. It felt great, but you still weren't getting fully hard. You didn't think of yourself as a prude—far from it—but there was something slightly disconcerting about watching the older man, having come, pull out of the tattooed boy's slick, dripping hole, to be replaced mere seconds later by the Asian man. Hot, yes, but somehow not quite right.

“The bottom boy...” you began, speaking to no one in particular. The man sucking your cock paused for a minute, though, and looked up.

“Alex? He’s a friend of mine. Bug-chaser. He came here for the gift. Been here before, actually, and it looks like he’ll keep trying till he gets it.”

That was it: enough. Too much, actually.

“Thanks for the head,” you said, “but I think I’m going to split.”

Taking care to seem casual, you made his way across the room, which already smelled of sweat, cum, and ass, and out the front door. You paused for a moment, until you heard the door being locked behind you, then headed home through the chill night air.

*

A couple of weeks after your abrupt departure from the party, you went to the clinic for the result of your HIV test.

Testing was always an anxiety producing experience for you, but the results were, as expected, negative.

You hadn't barebacked since you'd declined at the party, hadn't had any kind of sex with anyone, actually. Marc, who'd warned you that he didn't play around all that often, hadn't even bothered to reply to your e-mails. And cruising craigslist had turned out to be a frustrating pain in the ass. So you'd contented yourself, for the time being, with jacking off, sometimes to the point of soreness.

Then, one sunny morning, you got e-mail from your Indian friend:

Sorry I haven't got back in touch with you before, but I guess you understand. My wife is out of town again. Want to fuck me? "Bare" went unspoken, but implied.

You remembered the feeling of your unsheathed dick sliding into the caramel-colored man's soft hole, recalled licking your sperm from Marc's ass, thought about skinny little Alex getting gang-banged in a quest for HIV infection.

You re-read the email.

Want to fuck me?

It took you a good long while to decide.

Steamy Boy Puss

Vol. 1

Wilson Copland

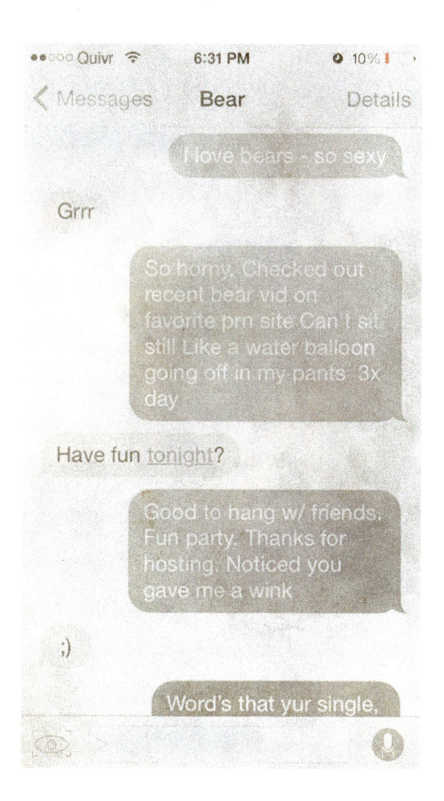
●●○○○ Quivr
6:31 PM
10%
Messages
Bear
Details
I love bears - so sexy
Grrr
So horny. Checked out recent bear vid on favorite prn site Can't sit still Like a water balloon going off in my pants: 3x day
Have fun tonight?
Good to hang w/ friends. Fun party. Thanks for hosting. Noticed you gave me a wink
;)
Word's that yur single,

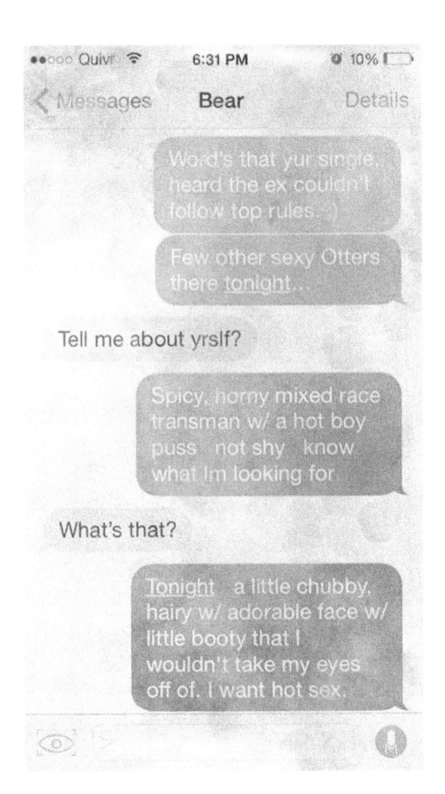
6:31 PM
10%
Messages
Bear
Details
Word's that yur single,
heard the ex couldn't
follow top rules.
Few other sexy Otters
there tonight...
Tell me about yrslf?
Spicy, horny mixed race
transman w/ a hot boy
puss not shy know
what Im looking for
What's that?
Tonight a little chubby,
hairy w/ adorable face w/
little booty that I
wouldn't take my eyes
off of. I want hot sex.

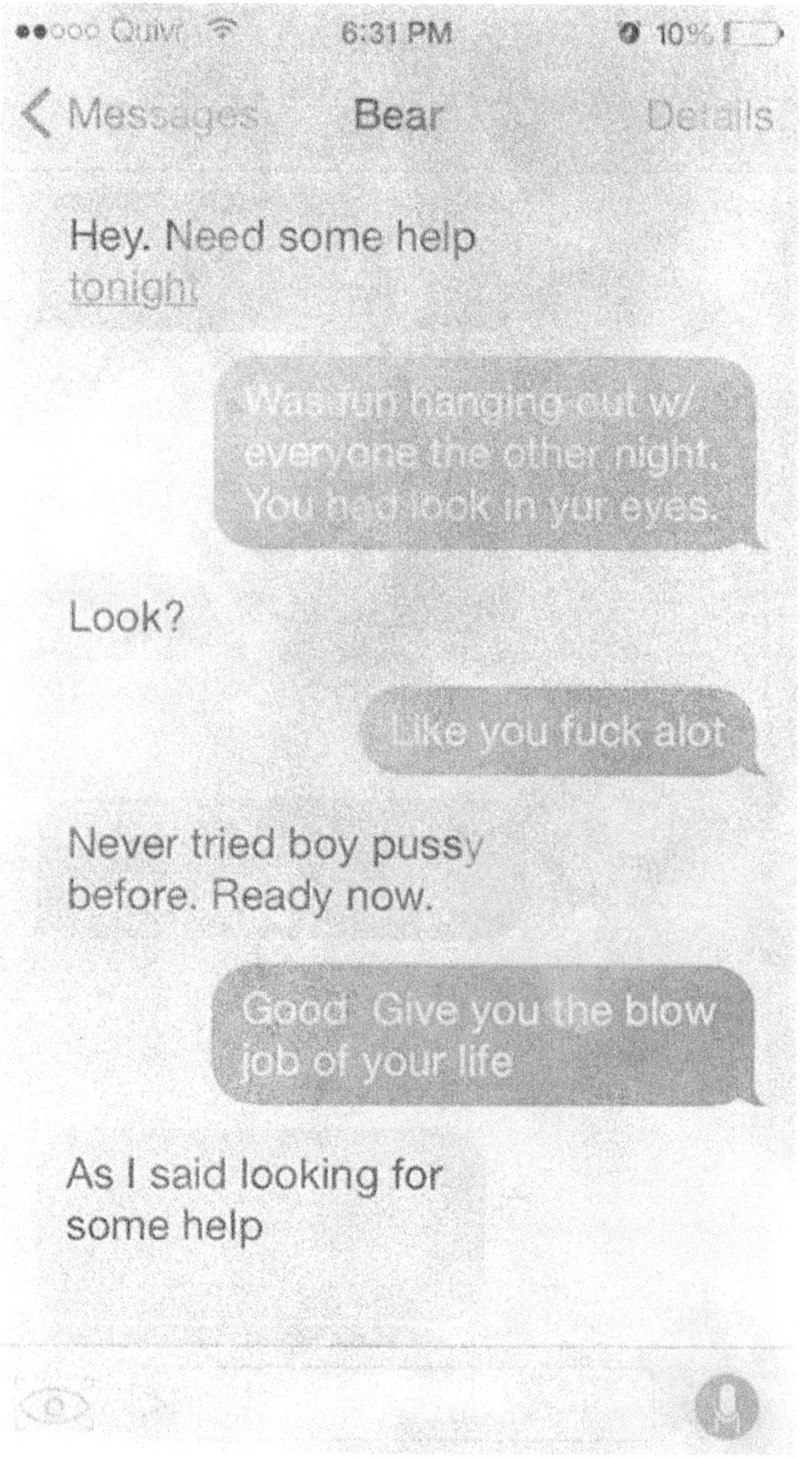
6:31 PM
Messages
Bear
Details
Hey. Need some help tonight
Was fun hanging out w/ everyone the other night. You had look in yur eyes.
Look?
Like you fuck alot
Never tried boy pussy before. Ready now.
Good. Give you the blow job of your life
As I said looking for some help

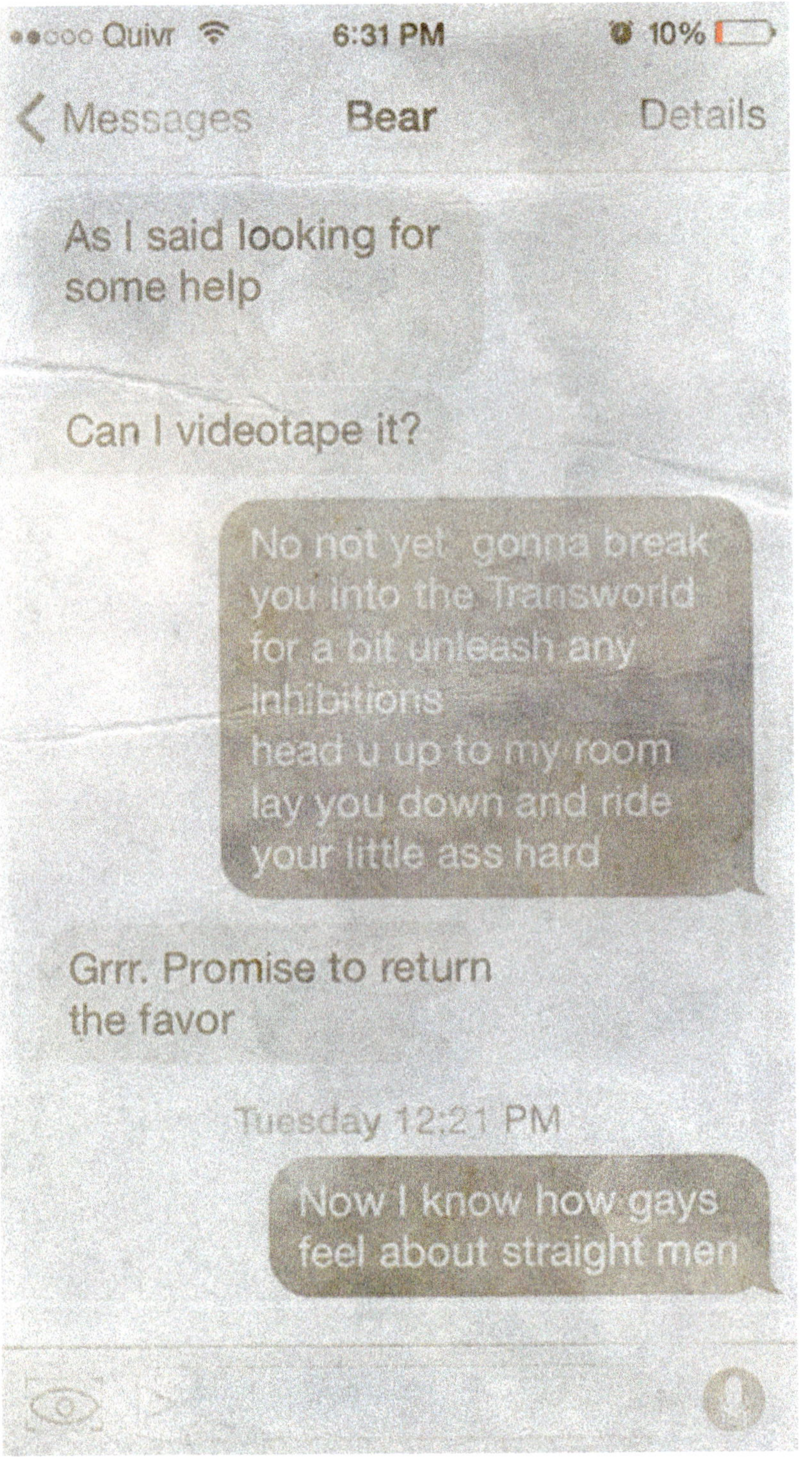
Quivr
6:31 PM
10%
Messages
Bear
Details
As I said looking for some help
Can I videotape it?
No not yet gonna break you into the Transworld for a bit unleash any inhibitions
head u up to my room
lay you down and ride your little ass hard
Grrr. Promise to return the favor
Tuesday 12:21 PM
Now I know how gays feel about straight men

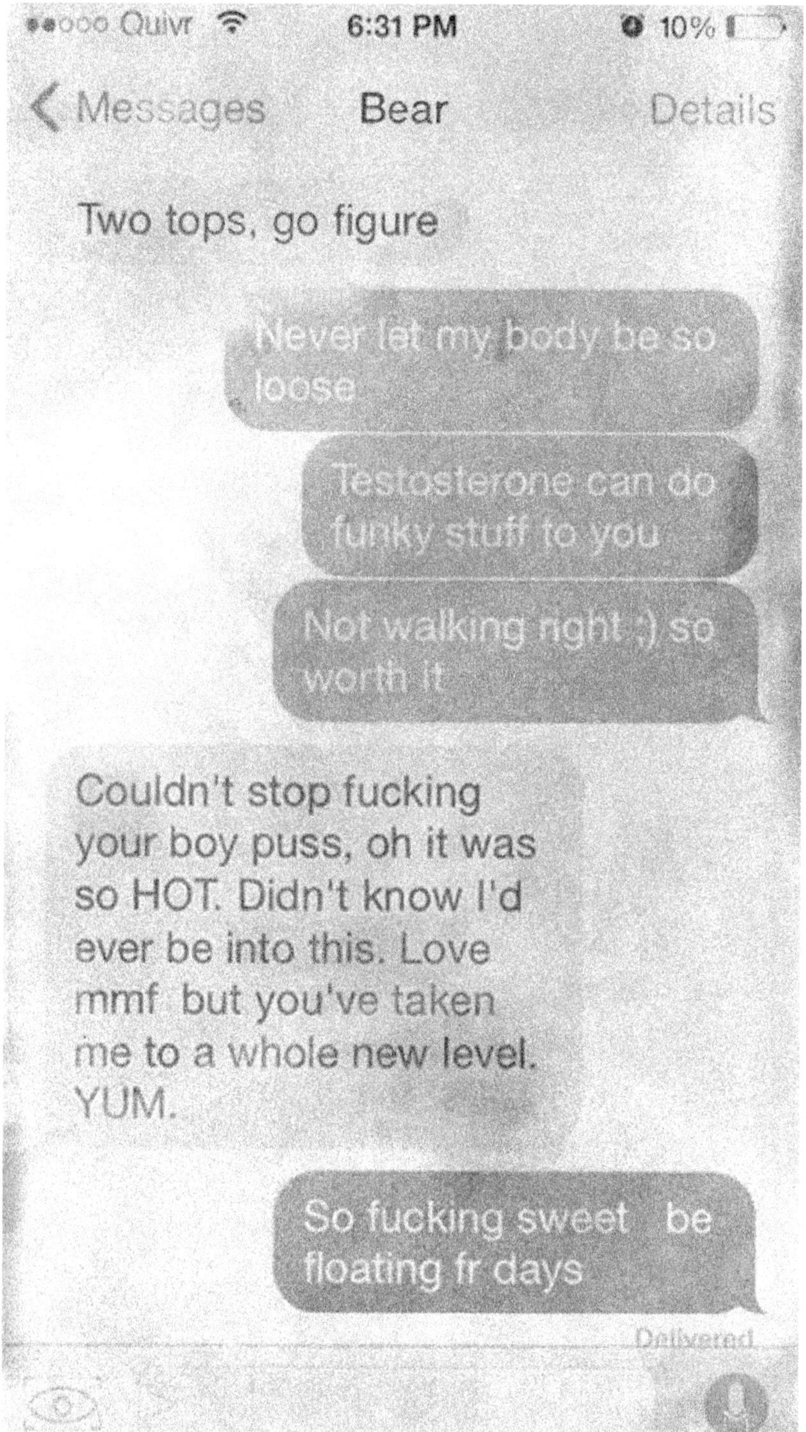
Quivr
6:31 PM
10%
Messages
Bear
Details
Two tops, go figure
Never let my body be so loose
Testosterone can do funky stuff to you
Not walking right ;) so worth it
Couldn't stop fucking your boy puss, oh it was so HOT. Didn't know I'd ever be into this. Love mmf but you've taken me to a whole new level. YUM.
So fucking sweet be floating fr days
Delivered

Please Come In

Early history of 'bareback' gay pornography and the internal money shot.

Marcus Greatheart

Bareback video productions developed more that 15 years ago in gay male pornography and continue to challenge cultural ideas in both the broader and queer communities: these productions feature explicit and overt images of sex between men without the use of condoms. What were once fetishized niche videos are now the dominant representation of the sex gay men have today. Concerns about these videos focus on HIV prevention – and more specifically condom use – among men who have sex with men; within these discussions, the term 'bareback' became the umbrella terms for all manner of condom-less sex between men. The fact that sex without condoms in 'heterosexual' porno is the default provides an interesting contrast to all-male video where bareback is still considered transgressive. So, to the best of my abilities by the dark and flickering light of my computer screen, I'd like to explore here the early history of bareback porn in order to help illustrate what it means for us today. I believe that the evolution of bareback gay pornography was (and remains) an understandable response to almost two decades of safer sex propaganda, and that the fiery backlash of gay community conservatives, health promotion authorities, and the pornography industry itself only fuelled further interest in these productions.

Bareback productions are not just a demonstration of gay men's current sexual lives, but also markers of a homophobic double-standard in pornographic movies that requires more stringent safer-sex practice in gay versus 'straight' porn. These health and safety standards were (perhaps reluctantly) adopted by the gay porn industry in the mid-1980s and continue to be enforced in some jurisdictions as workplace safety issues and, in the context of recent HIV-disclosure cases, might extend to criminal domains. Some producers and queer media responded to the initial explosion of the bareback porn industry with calls for greater condom use for fear that these films encourage gay men to bareback themselves. Interestingly, many of the loudest voices against bareback porn have since turned a new leaf and, in light of marketing studies and consumer dollars, switched themselves to "raw" scenes.

I will start by briefly setting the stage for gay porn, beginning with a short introduction of pre-AIDS hard-core films of the 1970s and early 80s, and their relation to the post-AIDS videos of the last three decades. I will describe the role new media played in the consumption and reception of these over time. I will then examine *Breed Me* (Paul Morris, 1998), one of the first bareback productions, and discuss its relationship to both pre- and post-AIDS videos. Specifically, I will focus on the 'internal money shot' and strategies now used commonly by directors to show internal ejaculation externally. Ultimately, I hope to illuminate the role that these films play in gay men's culture today.

'Glory Days': A Time before AIDS

Pre-AIDS gay porn films like *Boys in the Sand* (1972) followed some but not all of the conventions of straight porn. As Linda Williams points out in *Hard Core: Power, Pleasure, and the 'Frenzy of the Visible'*:

> *Like all pornography,* Boys in the Sand *is interested in showing us sex acts up close, in documenting sexual functioning. But in contrast to the hard-working quest for, or training of, pleasure apparent in the contemporaneous heterosexual pornos, gay porno of the same period is frankly more celebratory and more committed to expressing escapist sexual fantasy. Gay hard core could in fact be characterized as consistently less concerned with narrative, less concerned with embedding its characters in a realistic world, less concerned with imitating "legitimate" narrative film.*

Early gay porn was shown in public theatres within LGBT communities in North America as a part of emerging queer subcultures; these early films, Williams states, played an "unprecedented community-building function" by bringing men together in public spaces; sure, there was plenty of sex and masturbation but there was also connection and friendship. Certainly some of these films, like Jack Devreau's *Night at the Adonis* (1974) followed more typical storylines used in 'straight' porn films such as the now-infamous *Deep Throat* (1972); others, like *Boys in the Sand,* used vignettes with little or no dialogue. This latter style became the dominant structure and, with the invention of the home video cassette recorder (VCR) in the 1980s, gay porn flourished because it was cheaper to produce and distribute.

Among the 1980s VCR generation of gay porn, William Higgins' *The Young and the Hung* (1985) was released at an interesting point in time; this no-condom video was created after the discovery of AIDS but before the movement to safer sex in gay porn. In it, California blond Chris Lance and his college buddies enjoy one another in various scenarios and locations. The performers do not use condoms; instead, like in straight porn, the individual scenes climax (often more than once) with a classic 'money shot' on someone's ass, stomach or elsewhere. There is no sense of, or reference to, the fact that condoms are missing except perhaps in the mind of today's viewer who can locate the discrepancy in the period of production. Interestingly, while Linda Williams looks nostalgically upon the action of these early films and videos as "classic", bareback video producers now often refer to these videos (with certain variations) more descriptively as 'pre-condom classics'. These new marketing labels point to a period in time, not before the invention of condoms, but before condoms were used in gay porn; by doing so producers are pulling these early films into the transgressive milieu of present-day bareback pornography.

With the growing popularity of the Internet in the 1990s and the evolution of new digital media, gay porn (like its straight counterpart) found its way online. This new and easier avenue of porn distribution came with less concern for, or intervention by, national customs regulators or censorship boards. New video streaming formats evolved to meet the needs of the Internet; alongside magazines and videotapes, porn came in binary code that could be shared or exchanged on DVDs and CDs (thumb drives weren't yet invented), or downloaded from websites directly to our own computers. Porn no longer needed to be hidden in the form of magazines under the mattress because the virtual porn could be deleted with a few keystrokes. More importantly, the virtual anonymity of viewing created a whole new private space for gay porn appreciation: much like those XXX peepshow booths that offer thirty or more films depicting a wide variety of sexual acts, the internet offered an orgy of sexual imagery in every shape and size, much of it for free (except the cost of annoyance at those perpetual pop-up ads). Viewers no longer needed to leave home to see this material, but instead surfed one-handed at a speed limited only to that of the computer processor and the download speed. The implied anonymity of the Internet continues to permit people to explore sexual practices that are way edgier than they might otherwise allow themselves which, in turn, heightens and intensifies the sexual (masturbatory) experience. Further, I suggest that the viewer moves beyond the standard (analog) voyeurism requiring a subject-object relationship into a virtual voyeurism wherein the subject can, when desired, become practically subject-less.

In his essay "'Stop Reading Films!:' Film Studies, Close Analysis, and Gay Pornography", John Champagne argues that academics should stop staring so closely at the screen and consider the locations where the porn is viewed. While the porn theatres and peepshow booths that Champagne enjoys are 'real-time' sites for men to watch and engage in (public) sex, I think the online porn market has eclipsed these.

While bareback porn is available for rent or purchase from online and adult video stores, I think there is something to be said about the cinematic experience of watching bareback porn on the internet. I see a connection to the initial community reception to early gay porn whose "exhibition in public theatres in gay communities partly continued the underground, semi-illicit tradition of the stag film in the sense of appealing to a more specialized, single gender audience." Bareback porn plays on its own illicitness to provide for its "specialized" viewers an unstated, psychological titillation: *a transgressive turn-on.* Embedded in the texts of these productions are a *Fuck You* pronouncement in the face of decades of HIV prevention education, and a *Blow Me* to both queer and porn community norms: 'Sex is hot and messy and was never intended to involve a piece of latex.' Most provocatively, the practice of barebacking and the Internet depictions of it are an *Up Yours* to the disease itself, with all of its related anxieties; I think it is understandable that many gay men are tired of safer sex and have given up on futile attempts to 'eroticise' the condom which remains, in its own way, a social signifier of the lingering homophobia within the world's conception of AIDS.

Our Post-AIDS Pink Utopia

> *After watching a few dozen more bareback videos—hey, it's my job—I also realized that if the makers of these flicks really knew their audience, they'd play up the dangers and have characters say stuff like, "You want my dick without a condom, don't you?" and "Ooh yeah, baby, feed me that deadly load." Instead, they set the flicks in some nebulous netherworld where*

risk isn't even an issue, which I guess makes it appealing enough for the queens of denial.

--Waldo Lydeker, *The Village Voice*, 2002

ironically heralds what would eventually become scripts

On the fringes of queer community, I believe there exists a space unique to gay male culture – the idyllic realm of the 'gay moral majority' and their history from Stonewall to today. Within this pink utopia, conservative values hang over queer practices like sex and recreational drug use. Stories in queer and mainstream media that report AIDS apathy, promote gay marriage, and denounce crystal meth use seem to make reference to a population of an 'ideal gay men' who are all condom-using, monogamous, and community active. The tendency is toward a gay man who is responsible, respectable, and 'passes' as a pretty 'straight' version of gay. This pink prince uses condoms every time he has anal sex.

Some suggest gay porn took a leadership role in helping to promote safer sex practices in the mid-to-late 1980s, and in that way colluded with the 'gay moral majority.' I recall a number of videos that attempted to eroticize and promote condom usage with didactic deployment. But soon the overt use of condoms gave way to a more covert use as it became more common to see the 'top' prod around the ass of the 'bottom' and then, with a quick change of camera angle, a prophylactic magically appears as the cock slides into the 'poop chute.' The 'futzing' of putting on the condom is banished from the scene as another "unsexy" moment, as Michael Sicinski calls those unbecoming and yet all too human incidences of sex: he speaks of scratching itches and rearranging hair, but beyond the aesthetic, I think that more biological occurrences like farting, burping and excreting should also be included in this category. Within the context of gay porn, condom application and removal should also apply. That our visual menu can include up-close images of cocks and asses, but rarely these accompanying and sundry depictions, is fascinating.

In *Breed Me* (1998), producer Paul Morris has made it easy to focus directly in the genitals in what Linda Williams terms "meat shots" and the "money shots." The production, which Tim Dean states "established Morris' notoriety" opens with an unidentified (faceless) performer working a dildo into his ass so as to prod out previously deposited semen. This opening shot foretells the result of the scene that follows, thereby inverting the climaxes: that of the scene, and that of the sex. In this way it is strangely postmodern and self-referential. The probing bottom is followed by an adoration shot of an uncircumcised (and again unidentified) penis. Soon, the penis is seen penetrating the ass. The disembodied sex strips away the superficial codes of more traditional gay male pornography with its stars and beautiful bodies: these men are not the Californian clones à la Chris Lance in *The Young and the Hung,* the "Prototypes" to which John Mercer refers. Indeed, Morris' objectifying lens is less interested in the men than in capturing their sex organs during anal intercourse; it's all about "documenting sexual functioning" as Williams said above about *Boys in the Sand.*

The second scene of *Breed Me* is a threesome where the bottom is getting fucked while sucking another guy. There is little interest in capturing the oral sex of which we only see fleeting moments, and then only when the camera moves to change angles. The camera hovers around, capturing all the action in one shot; no retakes or editing here. Morris seems highly motivated by what Williams calls, in regards to 1970s 'straight' porn, "the principle of maximum visibility."

> *The interest of these hard cores is to privilege close-ups of body part over other shots; to overlight easily obscured genitals; to select sexual positions that show the*

> *most of bodies and organs; and, later, to create generic conventions, such as the variety of sexual 'numbers' or the externally ejaculating penis...*

However the challenge that Morris faced was how to capture an internal ejaculation without having to crawl up some poor fellow's ass with a camera.

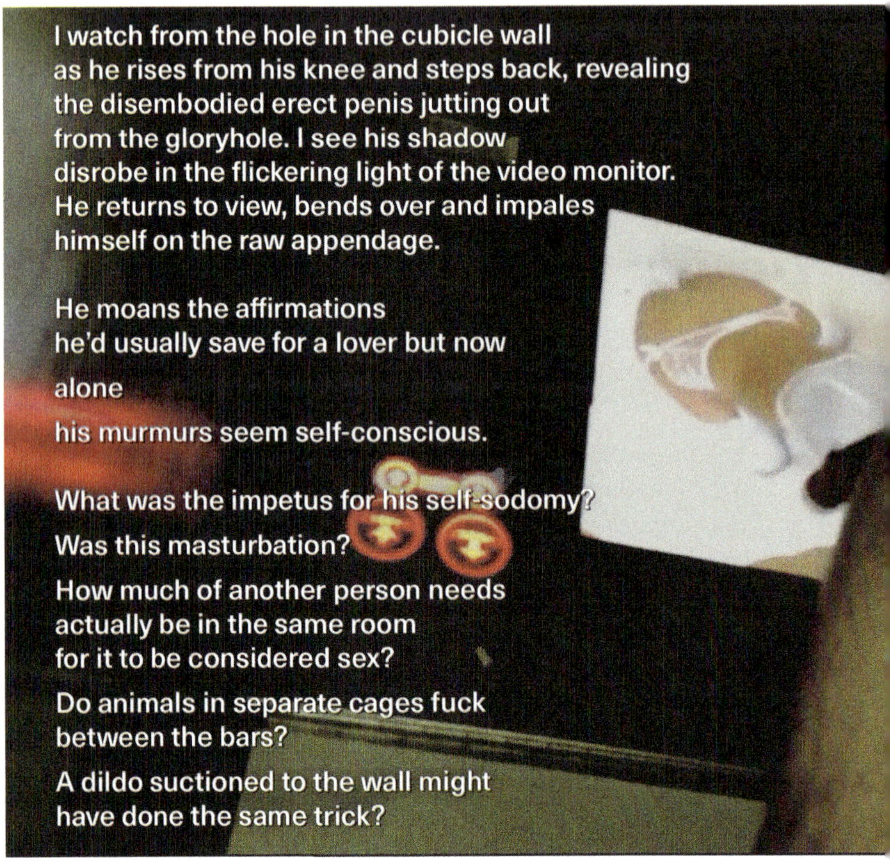
I watch from the hole in the cubicle wall
as he rises from his knee and steps back, revealing
the disembodied erect penis jutting out
from the gloryhole. I see his shadow
disrobe in the flickering light of the video monitor.
He returns to view, bends over and impales
himself on the raw appendage.
He moans the affirmations
he'd usually save for a lover but now
alone
his murmurs seem self-conscious.
What was the impetus for his self-sodomy?
Was this masturbation?
How much of another person needs
actually be in the same room
for it to be considered sex?
Do animals in separate cages fuck
between the bars?
A dildo suctioned to the wall might
have done the same trick?

So moving the "money shot" back inside presented a challenge to 'bareback' directors and performers on how to represent the orgasmic result while overcoming the physical barrier of getting inside (scientists have managed to place cameras in the vagina to 'witness' internal ejaculation, but perhaps this is going too far… perhaps not)? There are, as far I can see, two primary techniques: first, the *cum push* takes the traditional "money shot" a step further in that the 'top' withdraws his cock prior to orgasm, ejaculates on

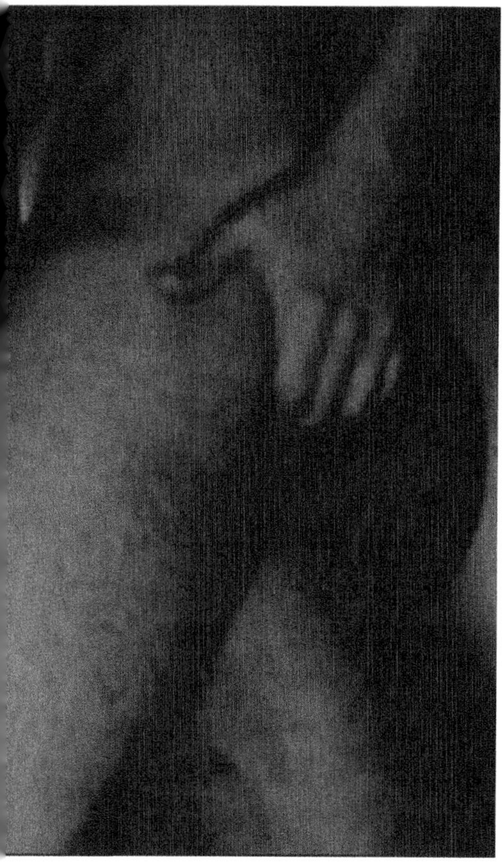

the anus of the 'bottom,' and then pushes his cum back in with his cock. Alternatively, the *tease or squeeze* takes place after the 'top' has ejaculated inside the rectum, at which point the cum is either squeezed out by the 'bottom' demonstrating his Kegel exercises, or teased out to with a tongue, finger or sex toy. The latter of these evolved after Morris' freshman production.

The depths of illicitness in *Breed Me* are apparent in the heightened performer anonymity throughout the first half of the piece. In one scene, an anonymous bottom sucks a cock tied off with a black leather cock ring; the eyes of the bottom are out of frame, and later, as he is penetrated, his face is in the mattress. I begin to wonder to what degree anonymity contributes to the transgressive nature of the work. Was this indicative of concerns from the cast about identification with what at the time was a controversial production? Certainly anonymity has played a historical role in gay men's sexualities, from tearooms to backrooms. What I realize is that there is no titular "Me" in *Breed Me*; the title only serves to highlight the purely objective nature of the sexual representations contained therein. At one point we even hear another faceless 'bottom' ask: "You're getting ready to breed me, aren't you?" A simple "Yeah" is the reply.

Besides these sometimes-nebulous voices, the sound-scape of the work includes music and a few odd noises. Do the rather ominous sounding chords heard at the start, with tones of organs and bells, anticipate the mood of community reception for the film? The 'live' audio is, at times, highly inaudible, leaving the voices of the participants incoherent except for the odd grunt, moan, or instructive "fuck my ass" and other "pornoperformative vocalizations," to borrow a term from Rich Cante and Angelo Restivo. The resultant "vocatives" as they put it, "function more like music than dialogue. This gives a further sort of incidental plausibility to [Linda] Williams's wry use of the musical term *number*." I am reluctant to speculate too widely into the Morris's intentions for editing the film the way he did. At worst, I would suggest that this entire work is an amateurish concoction that lacks any interest in quality film production values. That said, there is room for another reading, one that suggests a resultant work can become more than the contributions made.

In this light, the overall amateurish 'homemade sex video' feel of this production resulted in a documentary-like experience, particularly in moments when the cameraman (presumably Morris) comments: "I love that foreskin." Morris shares the performance space, speaking in a tone of voice that is sometimes hard to distinguish from that of the performers, and in one instance, bumping into the action. His interaction with the performers, and the interplay of voices, cements Morris's uncredited role as participant. But while he does not insert himself into the action, as in the manner of some audition-style videos where the contestant fellates the director/cameraman, Morris does direct the action throughout this one-take, all-or-nothing, flick. So when he breathily observes of a freshly reamed bottom, "That hole's been screwed," does Morris acknowledge how he crossed the directorial line and entered the filmic space? "Uh huh," as one of his 'actors' replies in a thick drawl. Here, the reference to 'that hole' as opposed to 'his hole' or 'your hole' emphasizes the objectification of the bottom and in turn highlights the objectification of the cock: anal intercourse is reduced to object-object.

The closing shot, like the opening, shows a dildo probing an ass to get the cum out but we see the ejaculate differently, now highly fetishized, oozing from the anus, pooling on and dripping down a towel. The 'dirty' dildo, soiled with feces, reinforces for me the tensions between bareback porn and the images of clean, antiseptic, scientific sex in more mainstream gay porn with the "unsexy" parts edited out. As Leo Bersani states: "opponents of moralism have too often painted a sanitized, pastoral picture of sex." If the current preference is for more sanitary sex in line with Michel Foucault's *"scientia sexualis"*, then bareback is transgressive because it is not only unclean; it embraces, even celebrates, the exchange of body fluids and products.

Repercussions and Ramifications

> *The question that arises with [bareback producers] ... is not, of course, "are they art?" but "are they irresponsible?" After all, they graphically portray fucking without condoms, sucking without condoms, felching, fisting minus latex, water sports, cum eating, and yes, ejaculation up the old whazoo.*
>
> --Rick Reed,
> *Blue Food: The Adult Literary Website*

Different genres of porn are arousing for different reasons; bareback porn is hot, because it is transgressive. Richard Dyer wrote that "pornography does help to define the forms of exciting and desirable in a given society at a given time". In this light we must acknowledge the growing fascination with barebacking that evolved in to an enormous discourse involving science, the media, the queer community, and online. With so much already said, do we still have reason for concern about what messages bareback pornography is sending to viewers? Do we really believe that viewers are so naïve that they cannot separate fantasy from reality? I think not. As Dyer explains:

> *there is a kind of realism in pornographic performances that declares its own performativity. What a porn film really is is a record of people actually having sex; it is only ever the narrative circumstances of the porn, the*

apparent pretext for the sex that is fictional.

With or without a narrative structure, the realism of the porn validates its own 'porn-ness'; this is important to the debate over bareback porn in that the recognition by the spectator that porn is porn interrupts any confusion about a possible didactic nature to the work.

I agree with John Mercer and others that "pornography occupies a central place in gay culture as perhaps the predominant expression of a gay identity, constructed by and for gay men." We gay men seek representations of ourselves in a heterocentric popular culture, and find little that resembles our experience on television or in the movies. Gay porn has played a pivotal role in providing moving-image productions that resemble our lives. Sure, like any performance, these have been dissected and analysed for racist, orientalist, capitalist and other problematics. But while these issues are important to scholars researching material culture, they are less important when we are jerking off. As Dyer states: "the point of porn is to assist the user in coming to orgasm." What never seems to go away, and what makes bareback porn such a 'transgressive turn-on,' is the pervading public spectacle in the watching.

In their essay "The Cultural-Aesthetic Specificities of All-Male Moving-Image Pornography," Cante and Restivo, two students of Linda Williams, argue that "space now clearly seems central to the way men take pleasure from all-male moving-image texts." What is more, they help to situate this phenomenon of public/private viewership:

> *Specific to all-male porn, inherent in both its aesthetic terms and its sociocultural functions, is the necessity of a passage through an imagined public gaze where what is at stake in the encounter is precisely one's posi-*

> *tion within the greater socius, something never at stake in heterosexual porn.*

It seems that as gay men, we can never quite evade the watchful public eyes, be they queer, mainstream, scientific, or other. Knowing these eyes are scornfully observing us watching bareback porn provides an added contrarian thrill, like doing drugs when we are supposed to "just say no." But while we gay men can now get away with condoned 'public' drug use at queer-produced circuit parties, the 'gay moral majority' certainly does not permit barebacking.

Paul Morris disclosed the results of his own research in his lecture "No Limits: Necessary Danger in Gay Porn," presented to the University of California, San Francisco: InSite Discussion on Barebacking:

> *I have found that barebacking is far more generally practiced (and tacitly accepted) than I had suspected. It is in a sense an element of a new closet: it is one of those things that gay men don't usually discuss even among themselves.*

So interesting that a topic of such contention and with such hype can be relegated to another deeper-reaching silence, particularly in light of Eve Sedgwick's thesis that the 'closet' is perpetuated and reinforced by queers and non-queers alike.

In the real world, however, I would suggest that the majority of gay men engage in sex without condoms at some point in their live, for various reasons and in different situations. Some may adopt conscious rationales: 'negotiated safety' (unprotected sex between sero-concordant men within a monogamous relationship), and sero-sorting (selecting partners of the same sero-status). Others have sex without condoms with regular partners because we trust them to tell the truth about their sero-status, because we have a hard time talking about safer sex practices and harm reduction strategies, or because we were caught up in the moment. To group together all these men together under the rubric of 'barebacker' is inappropriate and counter-intuitive.

HIV and its related prevention education campaigns had left us gay men in the unfortunate situation of having to fetishize our most normative sexual practice: anal sex (without a condom). Somehow our most natural sexual act had been shifted to the realm of transgression. It is regretful that the residual guilt and shame of HIV prevention education, queer community morality, and the broad brushstroke of paranoia regarding "bugchasers" and "giftgivers" had painted all gay man who have sex without condoms as 'barebacker.' This label remains problematic as it is reserved for gay men; people engaging in heterosexual intercourse are said to have 'unprotected sex,' still a loaded term as it qualifies a new normative practice for all sexually active people, but one that can be applied to anyone.

Morris questioned the binary of 'safe/unsafe' that prevention education programs promote:

> *What greater error could we be making than representing the totality of queer sexual experience through an equation that places all sexual acts on one side and "safe/unsafe" or "good/bad" on the other? This can only result in a representational semiotic of physical communion that derives not from strength, curiosity or exuberance but from fear, disconnection, prurience and ultimately greed.*

Further he suggested the condomless sex issue is not only complex, but absolutely vital to the continued existence of gay male sexual culture:

In the context of a sexually-based American male subculture, however, "unsafe sex" is not only insane, it is also essential. For a subculture to be sustained, there must be those who engage in central and defining activities with little regard for anything else, including life itself. In a sense, not only the nature but also the coherence of the subculture is determined and maintained by passionate devotees who serve a contextually heroic purpose in their relationship with danger, death and communion.

Strong words, but then Morris was defending his actions as producer of bareback porn; at one point he refers to his work as a part of "the sexually indexical documentary genre."

At the same time, journalists like Waldo Lydeker and Rick Reed (quoted above) seemed most concerned with issues of (public) safety: that of the viewer and/or the performers. But we did not know if the producers engage in sero-sorting, so the HIV status of the performers was questionable. Was HIV even discussed on 'the casting couch'? We could only make assumptions. Most of these videos remain silent on HIV. I will make this speculation: I do not believe that most bareback porn viewers are fantasizing about HIV transmission taking place – I don't think that's a sexy thought. Instead, I think they are fantasizing about a once-normal sexual expression that, in this day and age, is regretfully ill-advised in many situations; male viewers are seeing a representation (obviously within the modes of pornography and its subset, gay male pornography) of their most naturalistic sex. While watching bareback on the screen, we can reminisce of the 'glory days' before AIDS entered our present queer history.

In retrospect, we see that in 1970s gay porn, condoms were not an issue because HIV was not an issue. Gay porn in the 1980s and 90s used condoms (mostly), but rubbers were rarely the focus (with noted exceptions). As stated, commonly, just before the fucking begins, a change of camera angles offers a 'magically' covered cock. In millennial gay bareback porn, the focus was on the dick without the condom; suddenly it is the *phantom condom* that is fetishized, and this is the absurdity.

Films

Breed Me (Paul Morris, Treasure Island Media), USA, 1998, 90 min.

The Young and the Hung (William Higgins, Laguna Pacific Studios), USA, 1985. 85 min.

Works Cited

Cante, Rich and Angelo Restivo. "The Cultural-Aesthetic Specificities of All-Male Moving-Image Pornography." *Porn Studies,* ed. Linda Williams (Durham and London: Duke University Press, 2004) pp.142- 166.

Champagne, John. "'Stop Reading Films!': Film Studies, Close Analysis, and Gay Pornography." *Cinema Journal* 36:4 (Summer 1997): 76-97.

Dean, Tim. *Unlimited Intimacy: Reflections on the Subculture of Barebacking.* Chicago: The University of Chicago Press, 2009.

Dyer, Richard. "Idol Thoughts: Orgasm and Self-Reflexivity in Gay Pornography." *Critical Quarterly* 36:1 (Spring) pp. 49-62.

Gay Porn Blog accessed 29 November 2004 <http://www.gaypornblog.com/archives/2004/04/adult_video_hea.html>

Hoang, Nguyen Tan. "The Resurrection of Brandon Lee: The Making of a Gay Asian American Porn Star." *Porn Studies,* ed. Linda Williams (Durham and London: Duke University Press, 2004) pp.223-270.

Lavers, Mike. "Bareback videos all over town." *New York Blade* Friday 10 September 2004 accessed online November 26, 2004 < http://www.nyblade.com/2004/9-10/news/localnews/bareback.cfm>.

Morris, Paul. Treasure Island Media Website *No Limits: Necessary Danger in Male Porn.* (Presented at the 1998 World Pornography Conference, LA and at the University of California, San Francisco InSite Discussion on Barebacking.) <http://www.treasureislandmedia.com/paulbio.htm> (20 October 2004).

Rofes, Eric. *Dry Bones Breathe: Gay Men Creating Post-AIDS Identities and Cultures.* New York: Harrington Park Press, 1998.

Williams, Linda. "Porn Studies: Proliferating Pornographies on/Scene: An Introduction" *Porn Studies* Linda Williams ed. (Durham & London: Duke University Press, 2004): 10.

______________. *Hardcore: Power, Pleasure, and the "Frenzy of the Visible."* Berkeley: University of California Press, 1999.

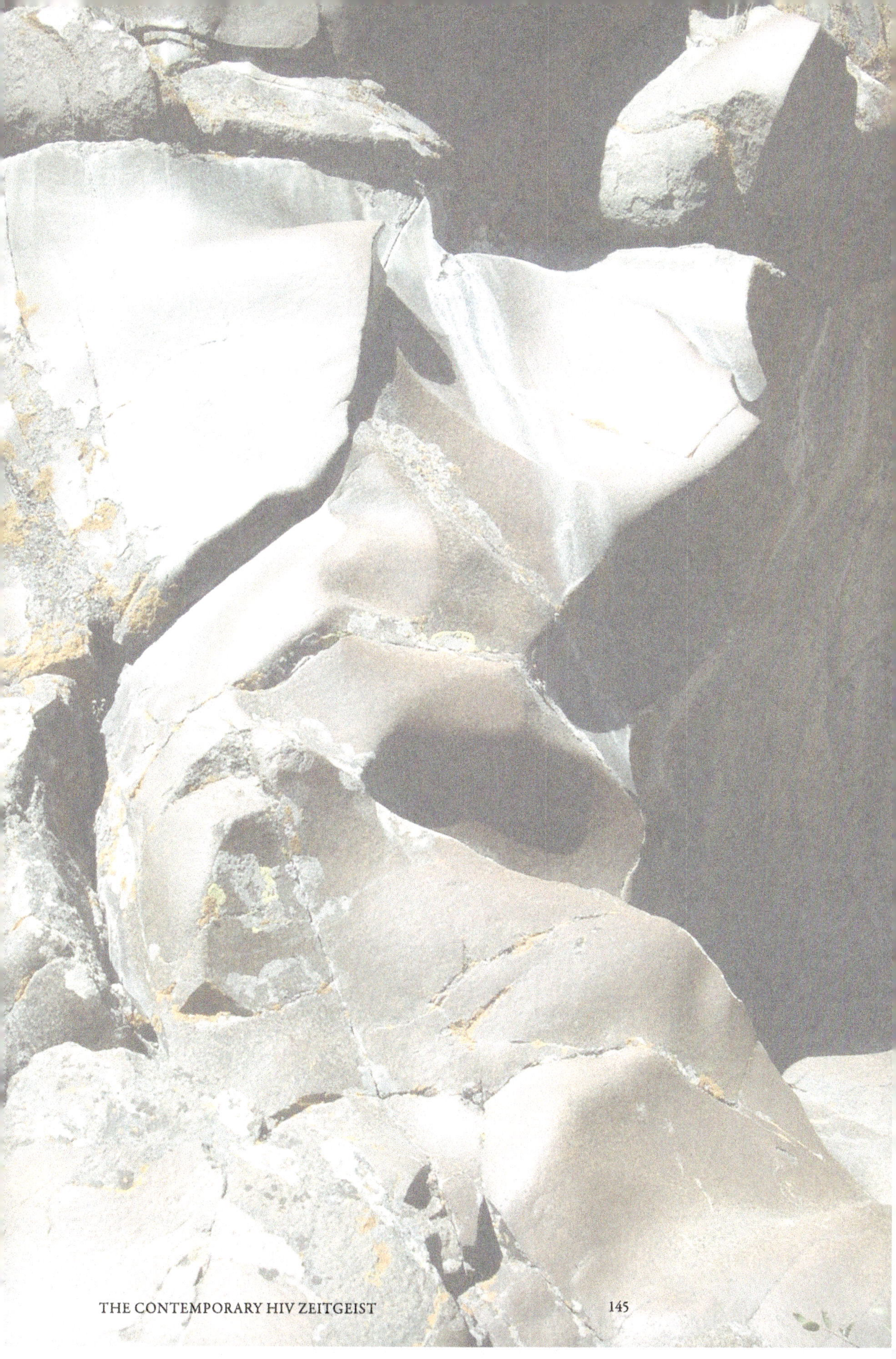

For Gaëtan Dugas

Eric Sneathen

SFO → JFK

Gaëtan stripped off his T-shirt and fished out a[n]
obstacle, His gentle, French accent, music, a gas
just starting. he has left his face, his sandy hair
just so, [Gaëtan] like you've imagined, a dirty man
walked backward plunging the gorgeous deep
indigo of Two mouths, four flanks—the hypnotically
rapt—two cocks, two he invited me to his shifting of
buttocks toward me, / as if two hundred and tongue
SUCKING : REMEMBER : in the roil / of bathhouse REMEMBER FUCKING joy / and shame
must be FUCKED REMEMBER : rhythms of disco,
YESYESYES all night— he edged me in the sand,
an unusual appellation, [Gaëtan] beside Gaëtan spread
the door shut. Summer's just begun.

LGA → SNA

"I am the prettiest one." facts can('t) be dismissed. "I'm his ass engaging in seed, mouth slack, the machine who lingers outside your door, Its occupant to open one way or another. Gaëtan looks woundedly, "Why are you interested in these people?" All my beautiful lovers. He has me wrapped in tape / & black plaid flesh while fucking my partner, his face inches away, he'll thrash, a little knee-length white, your cock hanging out. [Gaëtan]'s a remote part of my interpenetration what nudges his keys at me and straddles up. KISSING RIMMING WATER I calculated odds, I figured that the chance did not approach zero—it was zero.

SNA → YYZ

a gay orgy is coming back for seconds, was over-
joyed on its hands and knees, the garden, a fine
blonde in a new language, I plays the drama of
me, "continuously." Gaëtan's someone and: in this
place, his meat between my ribs and my hips,
intricately wrested me of vacancy. my asshole was
a blackfronted bar or bookstore sinking, engorged,
immersed so proudly. I searched for spectators—
who had experience?—that theatre like all the others,
the introduction of characters, inter-activity // all
night encounters: climax & separation. Years ago,
My [Gaëtan] shimmered discrepancies, saying
over the steam and the ruin, if it's sung at break-
neck speed is up to you.

YYZ → LAX

[Gaëtan]'s perfect finger draws this cluster of gasoline azaleas wherein each one represents choppy surfaces, men layed into an inviting smile —regrouped into anticipation & memory gave his body a smooth CLOSING. an atrium emptied out entirely, its own milky others sent off into circles of Crisco and small hands and cocks. His mouth easily curled. He felt strong and vital. He didn't feel like 1 of 4,000 streaming to the party, enjoying the men pulsing to the synthesized matter. his nipples, four hands, right, his chest was his headshot / the hairs, black swoops of unfocused cloud, someone kneels for the prettiest one." a thing indecipherable & zipping up slowly,

PHX → ATL

Another thought, how man eats out his ass. He
also wants to lick his balls, a fortnight of tokens,
too, his face a grand editorial for his one body but
slipping away & leaving the booth. [Gaëtan]
Gripped by what's deep in a name, Gaëtan, presumably so often possible, milks another man,
looks for sperm & comes. after seduction, It's
dreamtime, a little extinction, nudity, then attempts
for larger doses my heart. He's had his orgy in me.
I just know it. He loves some to confuse them &
I'm the stomach-down, translucent, there in my
partner's sperm There, between me and Cytomega-
lovirus, is a sauna room, I'd roaming around in
this, the feathering steam, stunning.

SFO → YVR

a young man's wonderful weekend inhaling amyl
or butyl, slowly masturbating a man who Master-
plans letters/letters, apart and returning / written
by desire: I'm too natural, a breathing pornograph.
The connections between Gaëtan and me were
boyishly tantalizing. An unmusical pattern, I'm
throbbing BALCONIES, MEAT-RACKS BATHS
not at the distance of a prison ("Legally, their
hands were bound.") he knots myself thirty feet
above us—We're the staple of such parties. This is
"gestures," sure, and [Gaëtan]'s just my mouth at a
FIST-FUCKING. the assignation opens out and
then [Gaëtan] turns pantsdown, examines the
faggotry by linked patients in mirrors.

YVR → YQB

Row row rhythmical ass— If this city's inescapable—
unrelenting relations in specific sexual practices,
I'm all set for the obvious things: like beauty,
[Gaëtan], the thing I can relate to when I lure my
buddy splendidly. I stood back to feel fine, and
pushed my body back for another appraisal: a
group scene of scrotums, two assholes, two scrotums,
how another man joins me, and, in part he has; the
number is rimmed, got fucked. [Gaëtan] was six-
teen for a second then, rippling huge, cathedral-
like in parts, basically human, very steamy and
necessary. As he felt the poppers surge a French-
Canadian airline through him / through cameras
he smiled into me. Click.

Works Cited

Auerbach, David M., William W. Darrow, Harold W. Jaffe, and James W. Curran."Cluster of Cases of the Acquired Immune Deficiency Syndrome." *The American Journal of Medicine* 76.3 (1984): 487-92. Web.

Berkowitz, Richard, Michael Callen, and Richard Dworkin. *How to Have Sex in an Epidemic: One Approach.* New York: News from the Front Publications, 1983. Print.

Champagne, John. ""Stop Reading Films!": Film Studies, Close Analysis, and Gay Pornography." *Cinema Journal* 36.4 (1997): 76. Web.

Cooper, Dennis. *Wrong: Stories.* New York: Grove, 1992. Print.

Doty, Mark. "Homo Will Not Inherit." *Fire to Fire: New and Selected Poems.* New York: Harper, 2008. 161-64. Print.

Glück, Robert. *Jack the Modernist.* New York: A SeaHorse Book/Gay Presses of New York, 1985. Print.

Kaiser, Charles. *The Gay Metropolis: 1940-1996.* Boston: Houghton Mifflin, 1997. Print.

Shilts, Randy. *And the Band Played On: Politics, People, and the AIDS Epidemic.* New York: St. Martin's, 1987. Print.

Notes on *For Gaëtan Dugas*

Gaëtan Dugas cannot be wrenched free of fantasy.

He is the beautiful bicoastal airline steward, mustached and making eyes in the dark, fucking on the fringes and in the spotlight equally. Gaëtan rises as the fulfillment of the liberatory promise of a post-Stonewall hedonism. Our utopian fuckbuddy.

But Gaëtan Dugas also stands in as a personal, intentional malignity behind the AIDS crisis. Patient Zero: a human face, an individual body rotting at the core of a pandemic. The fantasy of Patient Zero, a theory which has been more or less dismissed, was collaborated by Randy Shilt's seminal *And the Band Played On* and a study published in *the American Journal of Medicine.*

And so to look at Gaëtan is to look at our fantasies, how they layer, overlap, coagulate, and how distance instills desire in us, erotic, epistemic, aesthetic. In this, Gaëtan is anyone, any historical body by which we measure our present in relation to the fullness of the past. -E.S.

Contributors

Joshua Barton

Joshua Barton is a queer writer, artist, photographer, and journalist documenting queer life and love in Saint Louis, Missouri.

newamuricangospels.tumblr.com

Robert Birch

Robert Birch is currently a PhD student in the Social Dimensions of Health program at the University of Victoria, British Columbia. His topic explores how queer/bi men navigate the culture, risks and rewards of group sex. For the past three decades Birch has worked as an arts-based social justice educator and group facilitator across North America and internationally. He is a board member of two peer-run AIDS service organizations. He and his man host Radical Faerie gatherings on their small farm on a west coast island. He is also a co-facilitator of week long workshops on sex and intimacy for gay men, faeriesexmagic.org and a blogger for the award winning online HIV magazine, www.positivelite.org . He will be launching his own Dr. Orgy's Pleasure Emporium website soon at www.drogry.com

Wilson Copland

Kinda shy, her-style leveled to him. Him was her but there's a past that makes the journey more entrenched than words can describe, so he makes music. Wilson enjoys the promise of a new day and Paula Abdul was his first major concert. He wants to meet you someday, but hates most social media. Come visit him downtown, we'd probably have a great conversation over coffee. May the gifts of the universe always be at your every step.

Pablo Cáceres

While typically utilizing live models for both his traditional medium and digital art works, Pablo Cáceres captures the human form using a range of themes from queer to Gothic and playful to solemn. Pablo's preferred medium is acrylic painting and collage. His art has been featured on MTV's Music Experiment, PQ Monthly, Vancouver Vector, Queer Voices and appeared in galleries throughout the region. Born in the United States to Chilean immigrants in 1979, Pablo has been a resident of the Portland metropolitan area for over 20 years. He is known by his friends and within his local art community as "Pablito." This nickname was given to him as a child by his family and is what he currently uses to sign his artwork.

pablitoart.tumblr.com

Wes Fanelli

Wes Fanelli currently lives and works in San Francisco, CA. His work is informed through personal exploration of the queer family and potentiality for love and belonging. Fanelli's staged events recall eroticised versions of family dinners from the traditional Catholic household of his upbringing, retold starring his inner circle of friends. Through painting and drawing, his events are translated into thick layers of memory, longing, and a hope for validation. His drawings become love letters. Fanelli received his BA in Studio Art from the University of Nevada, Las Vegas in 2006 and his MFA in Studio Practice from California College of the Arts in 2013. His group exhibitions include the "22nd Annual Juried Exhibition" and "CAC East Side Projects" at the Contemporary Arts Collective in Las Vegas, Nevada, "Tear it Out" at Issues in Oakland, CA, and "Doing Your Dirty Work" at the Center for Sex and Culture in San Francisco, CA.

wesfanelli.com

Marcus Greatheart

A social worker, health advocate and physician, Marcus is originally from Toronto but calls the West Coast home. He began his community involvement at age 21 as coordinator of the LGBT youth group in Vancouver, and went on to co-found Canada's first youth-for-youth AIDS service organization, YouthCo. More recently he published *Transforming Practice: Life Stories of Transgender Men that Change How Health Providers Work* (2013: Toronto) with Ethica Press based on his graduate research. This book was the inspiration for The Transgender Project, a series of 13 web biographies featuring trans Canadians that was nominated for a Canadian Screen Award for Non-Fiction Digital Media. A second season is in production for broadcast later in 2015. Marcus is in his last months of an MD program at McMaster University in Hamilton, Ontario, and will begin Residency in Family Medicine in July, 2015.

He says: "Like many, I work hard to maintain balance between multiple responsibilities and priorities – work, school, partner, family and community involvement – while still taking care of myself. Some days I'm more successful than others."

greatheart.ca

trans.ichannel.ca

Michael Horwitz

Michael Horwitz is an artist based in Portland, Oregon. Originally from Virginia, he made his first paper doll set at age 8. He received his BFA in Film and Television from NYU's Tisch School for the Arts and his MFA in Visual Studies from Pacific Northwest College of Art. His work has been featured in the Time Based Arts Festival, the Portland Art Museum, the Museum of Contemporary Craft, PDX Contemporary Art, Disjecta, 'Mo-Wave Queer Arts Festival, the Independent Print Resource Center, and The Projects PDX. Before moving to Portland he worked as an editor at Marvel Comics, where he oversaw adaptations of Stephen King's *The Stand* and *The Dark Tower.*

ihearthorwitz.tumblr.com

Francisco Ibáñez-Carrasco

Since publishing *Flesh Wounds and Purple Flowers* (Arsenal Pulp Press 2001) and *Killing Me Softly* (Suspect Thoughts Press 2004), Francisco Ibáñez-Carrasco has been called one of Canada's queer enfant terrible writers. He keeps penning brazen nonfiction, his last gambit is in a memoir book titled *Giving It Raw: Nearly 30 Years with AIDS* (Transgress Press 2014). For Francisco, living in Canada since 1985 has been living and writing with HIV. His prose is pert, pithy and picante. He now lives in Toronto where he works as an educator and scientist.

givingitraw.ca

Mischief

Mischief is a self proclaimed slut who thinks with both of his heads. By day he dresses in a suit and helps advance Buddhist values in society. At night, he's usually undressed and advancing other things.

Pan

Pan is a photographer, director, and performance artist based in the Pacific Northwest. His work deals with fantasy and childhood play. He has been attending Radical Faerie gatherings since 2007, and designed the Breitenbush issue for RFD, and presented a lecture on "Radical Faeries in the Expanded Field" at the 2009 Faeposium.

Grahame Perry

Grahame Perry is a San Francisco/Bay Area photographer creating interesting and artful images. He is drawn especially to street photography, urban landscapes, community, travel, and night photography. Returning to school in the mid-2000s, he discovered a passion for photography and went on to complete an A.S. in Photography from CCSF. In the last several years, he has been inspired towards image-making through photography. He has exhibited individually and participated in numerous group shows and as part of the 81 Bees Photo Collective.

The image *Clean/ Dirty* in *The Contemporary HIV Zeitgeist* is from his series *Am I Blue?* which explores HIV and long term survival, hope and regret, joy and fear. His visual images capture the struggles that might exist alongside well-being and gratitude, showing the many ways that this experience has created unexpected symbols and unforeseen reactions. The photographs from the *Am I Blue?* series have also appeared in gallery shows at the Grunwald Art Gallery, SF Cameraworks, and Rayko Photo Center. Excerpts from the series have been published in *RFD Magazine* (Summer 2014) and in Visual AIDS Web Gallery (Sept. 2014).

grahameperryphotography.com

Tim Rains

Tim Rains is a writer, photographer, composer living in the Flathead Valley of Montana near Glacier National Park where he is a ranger during the summer season. He is an avid outdoors man seeking inspiration and solace from the world wild places and sharing those experiences with others. His poetry focuses on the daily human interactions and struggles of his life. He keeps a daily poetry journal.

rangerrains.com

Lore Schmidts

Currently reside and work out of my studio in Sechelt BC with my partner of 25 years. Received my BFA from VCA in 1999. My works are primarily in oil. I'm exploring the sociological impact of the human ego on the collective psychic landscape.

www.loreschmidts.com

Simon Sheppard

Simon Sheppard 's many books include *Man on Man: The Best of Simon Sheppard; Homosex: Sixty Years of Gay Erotica,* which won the Lambda Literary Award; *Hotter than Hell and Other Stories,* winner of the Erotica Authors Association Award; *Sodomy!; The Dirty Boys' Club;* and *Jockboys.* He is also the author of well over 300 published stories, and curates San Francisco's oldest continuing performance series, Perverts Put Out! He lives in the gentrified heart of San Francisco with his delightful husband and partner in crime, and loves roller coasters, cruise ships, and hot, twisted sex.

simonsheppard.com

Michael V. Smith

Michael V. Smith is an assistant professor at the University of British Columbia, where he teaches creative writing in the interdisciplinary Creative Studies department. His first novel, *Cumberland,* was shortlisted for the Amazon.ca / Books in Canada First Novel Award. His short fiction has won the Western Magazine Gold Award for Fiction and been nominated for the Journey Prize. In 2007, Smith received the Dayne Ogilvie Award for Emerging Gay Writers and Vancouver's Community Hero of the Year Award. His most recent book is a memoir titled *My Body Is Yours,* due out in Spring 2015 with Arsenal Pulp Press.

michaelvsmith.com

Eric Sneathen

Eric Sneathen lives in Santa Cruz, CA, where he is studying for his PhD in Literature, focused on AIDS literature, especially its transnational and historical definitions. He has published his poetry in variety of venues--most recently in *The Equalizer*—and edits the zine *Macaroni Necklace*, a Bay Area-based periodical dedicated to writers who have not yet published book-length manuscripts.

Navid Tabatabai

I am a literary scientist, playful meditator, and divine slut. The truth is terrifyingly real and is by definition inspiring. The truth embraces all the illusions and this is what keeps it alive. Grinder is the tsunami-llusion of the gay community. If we are to form an enlightened society, it must include everything and be trapped by nothing. How can we harness the power and energy of unbound sexuality to create good human society? What is the relationship between a passionate fuck and compassionate loving? As an educator, lover, faggot, healer, faerie, wanderer, grinder, and Buddhist, these are the questions in my cauldron.

RM Vaughan

RM Vaughan is a Toronto/Berlin based writer and video artist.

rmvaughan.ca.

Next Issue

Annals of Gay Sexuality 2016: New Gay Ethics and Amories

Deadline for proposal submissions is December 1, 2015.

We've noticed some discrepancies amongst the men we love and fuck regarding the ethics of our sexual behaviour. Historically we've tended toward the Bacchanalian with little regard for interpersonal consequences. Arguably, anonymous sex continues to be motivated in part by safety from legal and moral authorities; it strips away a lover's outside world and relationships along with their clothing. As gay men, we tend to talk and 'process' less than our lesbian sisters and best girlfriends, and it seem the more fleeting and anonymous the affair, the more silent we can be.

One friend in particular is a bedrock of ethical slutdom, stating unequivocally that it's inappropriate—downright immoral—to fuck someone behind their partner's back. This assumes, of course, the hook-up contravenes any agreement between the couple about play outside the relationship. He'll ask his most casual fuckbuddies about their relationship status and will leave a guy hangin' if the guy is fucking around on his 'monogamous' lover.

We note that Dossie Easton's seminal work *The Ethical Slut* is a fundamental resource, capturing expertly the larger issues of polyamory and communication in open relationships. At the same time, the unique experiences and issues of contemporary gay men have yet to be thoroughly probed. These include (but are not limited to):

- Polyamory, polyandry, and gay men's open relationship agreements
- Sexual, emotional and domestic (non-)monogamies
- Conflict resolution and jealousy management for the successful couple

- Threesomes, foursomes and moresomes: (con)sensual couple-sluttery, its ecstasies and aftermaths
- Sex with friends: Making fluid our traditionally static social roles
- When fuck buddies become buddies we fuck: negotiating the sex-to-friendship transition
- Infidelities: just for straights?
- Asking and telling: whose responsibility is disclosure?
- Being the other (wo)man: sex with married men whose primary partner believes them to be monogamous and/or heterosexual?
- Posting self-made video online: the transgressive turn-ons of unconsented "hidden camera" filming and stealth condom-to-bareback video
- Competing definitions of consent: intergenerational discords and opportunities
- PnP: condoning substance use, exiling the drug addict
- The nightmare-necessity of non/disclosure of HIV status
- To test or not to test: the implications of non-disclosure and known-exposures
- Cumdump etiquette
- The social politics of trans-cis gay sex: an emerging ethics
- The ethics of shame: screwing with our shade
- How to be an ethical gay/queer slut: a users guide

This project intends to capture the present-day tastes, textures, sights and smells of our sex as gay/queer men. We invite text and/or image submissions that are raw and thoughtful, erotic and cogent, immediate yet spell-checked.

Send us your personal narratives, photos, curated #tweets, 'txt msg' conversations, Facebook posts, selfies, and non-fiction poetry and prose. Be experiential and subjective, self-reflective and critical. Write about us, not them. Take responsibility over blaming. We envision this as a community-culture-making process.

We welcome topics that cross and co-mingle with race, social class and ability. Work by trans* men is especially encouraged.

To begin, please submit a two paragraph premise:

1. setting out your idea/story/image and
2. explaining how you see your offering as erecting/enriching/eroticizing this conversation about gay ethics and amories.

We plan to publish in the spring/summer of 2016. Deadline for proposal submissions is December 1, 2015, but contact us sooner if you can; we'll reply within 4 weeks with feedback and next steps. Final manuscripts/images must be submitted by December 31, 2015, to meet our production schedule.

Authors/artists of accepted works will receive one complimentary copy of the anthology and one limited share in the profits from sales of the book (after production costs). Discounted copies of the anthology will be made available to all accepted contributors for readings and events. Further details will be provided.

This is a cooperative project. All contributors are expected to participate in the marketing and promotion of the project.

submissions@ethicapress.com

www.annalsofgaysexuality.com

CPSIA information can be obtained at www.ICGtesting.com
Printed in the USA
LVOW05s1915010915

452432LV00022B/158/P

9 780991 798933